Advance Praise for
Behind the Murder Curtain

"As if being hospitalized wasn't traumatic enough, spend some time with the ultimate wolves in sheep's clothing—medical professionals who murder the very people they're tasked with keeping alive. *Behind the Murder Curtain* is a nonstop thrill ride with Special Agent Bruce Sackman, who tracks and brings these killers to justice."

—TERENCE WINTER, creator and executive producer
of *Boardwalk Empire*

"Special Agent Bruce Sackman looks *Behind the Murder Curtain* and doesn't like what he sees. Then he does something about it. An amazing look into a scary world."

—NICHOLAS PILEGGI, author of *Wise Guys* and *Casino*

"Everyone who reads *Behind the Murder Curtain* will experience an epiphany about the dangers that lurk within the presumed secure environment of hospitals. For two decades Bruce Sackman has been educating nurses about medical serial killers to improve early detection of unspeakable crimes. Bruce Sackman's shocking revelations about healthcare workers, disguising themselves as merciful caregivers, who murder their patients is a must read for forensic nurses. The motives, the murder plots and their execution masterfully unfold in this true crime story that reads like a novel."

—JANET BARBER DUVAL, MSN, RN, FAAFS, forensic nurse
educator and consultant, co-author *Forensic Nursing Science*

"*Behind the Murder Curtain* shines a light on a macabre world where we are betrayed by people we trust the most. Special Agent Bruce Sackman's groundbreaking work to bring down medical serial killers is the stuff of great detective novels but more frightening because it's true. This book may keep you awake at night but it is worth a nightmare or two."

—RUPERT HOLMES, multiple Tony and Edgar award-winning author of Broadway's *The Mystery of Edwin Drood* and Nero award-nominated Best American Mystery Novel *Where the Truth Lies*

"When patients at a VA hospital are dying at an alarming rate, Special Agent Bruce Sackman is called in to find out why. What he finds *Behind the Murder Curtain* is the stuff of great detective fiction…but it's true!"

—OTTO PENZLER, owner of New York's Mysterious Bookshop and editor of *The Big Book of Jack the Ripper*

Also by Jerry Schmetterer

The Godplayer: The Story of Pool Champion Bruce Christopher
The Coffey Files: One Cop's War Against the Mob
*The King of Clubs: The Story of Scores—the Famous Topless Club
and the Lurid Life Behind the Glitter*
E-Man: Life in the NYPD Emergency Services Unit
*Crooked Brooklyn: Taking Down Corrupt Judges,
Dirty Politicians, Killers and Body Snatchers*

Also by Michael Vecchione

Friends of the Family: The Inside Story of the Mafia Cops Case
*Crooked Brooklyn: Taking Down Corrupt Judges, Dirty
Politicians,
Killers and Body Snatchers*

Short Stories by
Michael Vecchione and Jerry Schmetterer

*Hand of the Killer: How a Bloody Handprint
and a Baby's Pacifier Nailed a Killer*
Murder On the Bridge: From the Files of Mike V.

BEHIND THE MURDER CURTAIN

SPECIAL AGENT BRUCE SACKMAN HUNTS DOCTORS
AND NURSES WHO KILL OUR VETERANS

**BRUCE SACKMAN, MICHAEL VECCHIONE,
AND JERRY SCHMETTERER**

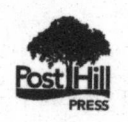

Post Hill
PRESS

A POST HILL PRESS BOOK

Behind the Murder Curtain:
Special Agent Bruce Sackman Hunts Doctors and Nurses
Who Kill Our Veterans

ISBN: 978-1-64293-538-7

Cover art by Cody Corcoran
Interior design and composition by Greg Johnson, Textbook Perfect

Post Hill Press
New York • Nashville
posthillpress.com

Published in the United States of America

DEDICATION

*To Eileen, Allison, Jonathan, and my grandchildren,
Brianna and Taylor, who fill me with joy
whenever they are near.*
B.T.S.

*To Lenor, Andrew, Brian, Suzanne, and the newest addition
to our wonderful family, Charles Nicholas Vecchione.
You are my world. I love you all.*
M.V.

To Dave and Minnie
J.S.

SPECIAL DEDICATION
TO AMERICA'S VETERANS

Working on this book reminded the authors of the debt we owe to our fathers, brothers, uncles, aunts, cousins, next-door neighbors, teachers, and just about anyone else who touch our daily lives and have served in the US Armed Forces. America's veterans set the gold standard of self-sacrifice and love for others. It is our duty to remember them, to serve them in times of need and to always hold them close in our hearts. We dedicate *Behind the Murder Curtain* to all veterans and single them out as examples of the best America has to offer.

Bruce Sackman: My father, Allan Sackman, who fought with the Third Armored Division at the Battle of the Bulge and my father in law, Ben Broder, who fought in Burma but never bragged or complained about their sacrifice for our country and always inspired me to follow their lead.

Michael Vecchione: Always on my mind throughout the writing of this book was my dad, a member of the greatest generation, Bronze Star recipient Private First Class Armando Vecchione of the 104th Infantry Division, US Army. He provided the inspiration that made writing this book a labor of love.

Jerry Schmetterer: I hope this book reminds our readers that despite its flaws, the people of the Veterans Administration, from orderlies to surgeons, are dedicated, conscientious professionals who every day serve those who served us so admirably. I am reminded of my uncle Benjamin "Bernie" Sacks who died at the Battle of the Bulge before I ever really knew him, and my brother Bernie who served with great honor in the war of our generation.

TABLE OF CONTENTS

AUTHORS' NOTE

This book is a result of more than three decades of Special Agent Bruce Sackman's service to the Veterans Administration. The main source of the material is Sackman's own notes, memories, and previous writings. It is complemented by interviews with his teammates in the battle against Medical Serial Killers. *Behind the Murder Curtain* also draws on public records, including court filings, newspaper and magazine articles, and a vast amount of information about the infamous characters depicted that is available in many forms to the reading public.

Bruce Sackman, Michael Vecchione, and Jerry Schmetterer

FOREWORD

When I first met Special Agent Bruce Sackman, I was the forensic pathologist for the New York State Police in Albany, New York. He traveled up from New York City because he had concerns about a young doctor who was suspected of killing patients in a Veterans Administration hospital. The doctor was currently in jail on fraud charges related to his obtaining a psychiatric residency at the VA Medical Center in Northport, New York.

Bruce explained to me that he wanted to use the time before the doctor was released to evaluate a possible murder case against him. He had no idea how many patients might have been murdered or how he would go about proving or disproving this theory. I had been involved in investigations and exhumations when there were sudden, unexplained increases in hospitals of unexpected deaths of relatively healthy patients.

Bruce was not a doctor. He seemed a bit overwhelmed by the task at hand. He had no experience in this type of investigation; he had no medically experienced support among his staff; and his bosses were not totally enthused about the VA's Office of Inspector General getting involved in murder. But I was impressed by his enthusiasm, his determination to do his duty as he saw it, and to charge the doctor criminally if warranted. He knew he was out on a shaky limb. I told him that the reason we do autopsies is because doctors and police can make mistakes in conclusions as to causes of death. I told him I would be glad to help.

The Hippocratic Oath is one of the oldest documents in history. Although written in antiquity, doctors hold its principles sacred to this day. The American Medical Association's Code of Medical Ethics holds that "the Oath of Hippocrates has remained in Western Civilization as an expression of ideal conduct for the physician." Above all, the physician should do no harm to the patient. Sadly, however, during my many years as a medical examiner, I have encountered a number of doctors, nurses, and other medical personnel who have intentionally done harm to their patients—who have murdered the persons in their care.

Unfortunately, patients in Veterans Administration medical centers have been the victims of some of these murders. Heroes who have survived war in far-off lands return home only to be killed by doctors and nurses assigned to give them comfort and make them well. If Special Agent Sackman wanted to do something about it, I wanted to help. Especially, because I had previously identified serial murders in civilian hospitals where the hospital administration did its best to help identify who did it, then discharged that person without charging him or her criminally, so that neither the family nor the public ever knew what happened. As a result, there would be no lawsuits, no bad publicity for the hospital. Bruce was clear—he wanted the perpetrator to be punished—and lawsuits and bad publicity be damned.

To identify that a medical serial killer (MSK) is at work, to conduct the painstaking investigation necessary to gather evidence against him or her, and to see to it that there is a

conviction and punishment, are not easy tasks. To be successful, it takes a special person leading a special team of dedicated, hardworking, and caring law enforcement and medical
professionals. Bruce is that kind of person and *Behind the
Murder Curtain* is his story.

Over the years, I have seen the results of the worst in
human behavior. I have examined countless numbers of dece-
dents to determine the cause and manner of death. In homicide cases ascertaining cause of death is often routine—death
by gunshot, by stabbing, by strangulation—and usually the
murder weapon is readily apparent. My findings have often
led investigators to the killer. The cases in *Behind the Murder
Curtain* were not typical murder cases. There were no obvious
causes of death, no murder weapons readily apparent, and
no clear perpetrator. These murders were committed behind
a privacy curtain in the secrecy of a hospital room by a lethal
injection where only the victim and his killer were present.
There was no obvious murder weapon—every patient in a
hospital has needle punctures from blood draws and intravenous fluid administration. The crime scene has been cleaned
by hospital personnel and the causes of death have initially
been attributed to the natural diseases for which they had
been admitted to the hospital, usually without an autopsy
being performed. Days, months, or years may have passed
before suspicions arose, usually caused by recognition of the
clustering of such unexplained deaths. The perfect murders.

Yet, remarkably, the murders were solved by Bruce and
his VA team, which also included FBI Special Agent Brian
Donnelly; a toxicologist; sound detective work; forensic medicine; and Bruce's Red Flags Protocol, a methodology he developed that is designed to catch MSKs. That system is now
used by law enforcement around the world.

Because of Bruce's work and his legacy, I say, MSKs beware! Hospital patients, whether in veterans' medical centers or civilian hospitals, you have a champion.

Doctor Michael Baden

Prologue

The young doctor with movie star looks, tanned and fit in a starched white doctor's jacket, stethoscope looped over his left shoulder, aviator sunglasses dangling from his pocket, sat in the hard chair about eighteen inches from his patient's bedside. They were alone, separated from the surrounding ward only by the thin curtain meant to offer privacy for the intimate interactions between doctor and patient. The only sounds were the mechanical clicks and beeps of the machines meant to monitor the life signs of the damaged men up and down the ward. The doctor sat for three hours, fixated on his patient, serenely watching the numbers on the monitor indicating the patient dying, dying, then dead. The doctor rose from his seat, made a notation on the patient's file, drew the curtain and went to the next patient on his rounds. A few minutes later, he reported to the nurse on duty that one of the patients in his care had unexpectedly died.

CHAPTER 1

The Adventure Begins

"Courage is knowing what not to fear."
—PLATO

My office, on the sixteenth floor of a bland government building adjacent to the Veterans medical center on Twenty-Third Street in Manhattan, was empty that day in May 2005 that I decided to pack up my personal property. My entire field staff was away for a week of training. There was no need for me to go because I would be gone when they returned. Retired.

So I was alone, sitting at my desk, which, like all the furniture in the building, was made by federal prisoners. I stared at the plaques and newspaper clippings on the walls. The clippings blared headlines that defined my career and my nightmares: *Angel of Death Killed 60, Mad Doctor Killed for Fun of It, Scientist Let Patients Die, Nurse Could Not Stop Killing.*

As a Special Agent in Charge of the Veterans Administration Office of Inspector General (VA OIG), I was responsible for the area ranging from West Virginia to Maine that

3

included 250,000 VA employees. I was retiring as a GS 15, the highest paygrade you can get in government service. Not bad for a guy whose friends called him the "nice Jewish kid from Brooklyn with a Glock on his hip."

VA OIG is a mouthful best explained as the office that investigates crimes that may have been committed against veterans and by employees of the Veterans Administration.

The preponderance of these crimes is nonviolent, like embezzlement, ID theft, petty theft of patient property, and fraud. They are crimes committed by aides, orderlies, clerks, pharmacy workers, and even nurses and doctors. People find it hard to believe that nurses and doctors may be criminals. We revere doctors in this country, and for the most part, they deserve our admiration and the rewards they receive. They save lives as commonly as a school crossing guard shepherds kids across the street. They enrich our lives and make us all better people for their efforts. And there are no people I admire more than nurses. They are the bedrock of our healthcare system. Without them, nothing gets done. And I found them to be the first line of defense against evil in the hospital wards.

That's the way I felt when I started this job in 1980 and that's the way I feel now. So you can imagine how reluctant I was to believe it, when I discovered about a decade ago, that there are doctors and nurses who purposely kill their patients. And when they killed, they killed in numbers that staggered the mind. I call them Medical Serial Killers (MSKs). as I filled a cardboard box with the mementos of my twenty-five years in VA OIG, it was the newspaper clippings headlined with the names Swango, Gilbert, Williams, and Kornak that slowed me down as I reread them. I remembered how I evolved from that nice kid from Brooklyn who investigated crimes that frankly were not challenging enough for me, into a homicide detective hunting doctors and nurses who killed for fun, greed, and misguided glory.

I was comfortable with my decision to retire. It was a financially sound one, and I was sensing a change in DC, where the current administration in 2005 seemed to be adding bureaucratic burdens, leaving less time in the field for investigations. My immediate supervisors down there wanted me to stay. Why not? I had put the VA OIG on the map with high-profile cases even though they were often embarrassing to the administration. I ran an efficient office. I created a team of nurses, scientists, medical examiners, and detectives who specialized in bringing down MSKs. But I was leaving things in good hands and would always be available as a consultant.

There was one piece of business to settle, however, before my caseload was totally clear. Doctor Paul J. Kornak was awaiting sentencing. A few weeks earlier, he pleaded guilty to criminally negligent homicide, making false statements, and committing fraud, in the death of an Air Force veteran named James DiGeorgio.

Kornak would be the last notch in my holster as a Special Agent. He was a different case than the other doctors and nurses I locked up for murder. He didn't kill for the thrill of it or to play God, as in my previous cases. He killed people because he needed bodies for a research project. He would enroll patients who did not meet the criteria of the project in order to keep his funding. He did not care what happened to them once they were a part of the experimental treatment. They were put at deadly risk because their medical conditions should have precluded them from being used in the experiment.

Kornak pleaded guilty to one count of criminally negligent homicide in the death of DiGeorgio. That's all the U.S.

Attorney needed but I was hoping he would push for more charges and even a charge of murder. I believed Kornak and an accomplice were responsible for several deaths.

Yet as evil as Kornak was, he was a choirboy compared to Doctor Michael Swango.

CHAPTER 2

Double O Swango

"When a doctor does go wrong he is the first of criminals. He has nerve and he has knowledge."

—SIR ARTHUR CONAN DOYLE
from *The Adventure of the Speckled Band*

In October 1995, I was just settling in to another day at the office, opening the file on an ongoing case, when Agent Tom Valery charged through my door and yelled, "Boss, pick up line one right now!" Tom was easily excitable so I didn't exactly drop the file I was reading and reached for line one. But when he continued into the room and took up position over my left shoulder, I sensed this call was out of the ordinary. I had no idea it would change my life forever. But it did.

"This is Special Agent Sackman," I said in my long practiced, measured "what is this about?" tone.

"This is Doctor Thomesen, I am a psychiatrist at Northport. You need to get out here right away. We have a doctor who is killing his patients," was the response. Without taking a breath, she told me something about a television show and a doctor named Swango. "How could this be happening?"

I had no idea what she was talking about but again in my long-practiced manner, I thanked her for calling and promised I would look into it. Without another word, she hung up. I sensed she was a little frustrated. I shrugged my shoulders, hung up, and looked up at Tom, who had been bent over the phone trying to listen in.

"I know what she is talking about," he said. "I think we should get out there. I'll give you a fill-in in the car."

It was not my style to rush into things. While I investigated crimes in VA medical centers and was trained to use the 9 mm automatic on my hip, my work rarely called for a lights-and-siren response. I was known for being skeptical and careful. Some thought I was bored, but believe me, I took everything in. I had heard many outrageous claims in my career, but never anything like this. Tom was an experienced agent and as he was already putting on his jacket and grabbing the car keys, I told my secretary I was going out to Northport and followed him out the door.

In less than fifteen minutes after the phone call, we were in the bare bones Chevy Caprice supplied by the Veterans Administration for use by its investigators, on our way to the Northport VA Medical Center. About seventy miles from our Manhattan office, we had both been there many times before on routine cases.

I chose to drive because I thought Tom was too aggressive behind the wheel and our rule was the driver controlled the radio. I liked Frank Sinatra and he liked Johnny Cash. As we bucked the heavy traffic, I looked across at Tom and asked if he thought there was really any merit to Doctor Thomesen's call? Of course, I wanted to ask him this as soon as I hung up the phone, but I did not want to dampen his enthusiasm, as he clearly had been eager to run out the door. The answer was typical in-your-face Tom: "Damn right, boss! Everyone in the office has been talking about the television show last night. It was about this doctor, Doctor Michael Swango. They said he served time for poisoning coworkers in Illinois, paramedics no less, and that wherever he goes, he leaves a trail of death. He's a resident at Stony Brook University Hospital in New York, practicing in Northport. The medical students call him "Double O Swango, Licensed to Kill" and "Doctor Death."

I asked, "The show said he killed people?"

"Well, they couldn't actually say that, but clearly they believe it and so does anyone who watched it," responded Tom.

Friends thought Tom and I were mismatched bookends. I'm a buttoned-down, conservative suit-and-tie guy who, I know, could pass for a Brooks Brothers salesman. I was a good listener and considered every move carefully; I tried to be the perfect image of an agent-in-charge. Tom, in contrast, was right out of a Damon Runyon story. He was old-school tough, quick with a joke, and disdainful of orders and anyone from "headquarters." In a dictionary, his picture would be included in the entry for "politically incorrect." We were about the same five feet, seven inches in height, but Tom was stocky and strong, the guy you wanted next to you in a foxhole. He was a volunteer firefighter in a town not far from where I lived, and many mornings he would show up to work after fighting a blaze all night. But together, our record proved we made a formidable team: I directed an investigation and handled "headquarters," and Tom followed his instinct and made noise when required (and sometimes when not required).

I drove on in silence. I was thinking about what I was getting into and how I would describe it to my bosses in Washington: "Doctor," "killer'. I was mostly concerned with white-collar crimes like embezzlement, identity theft, and, occasionally, pension fraud. I was pretty good at it. Once in a while, an investigation might involve missing drugs from a VA hospital pharmacy, and I would take part in a raid with the Drug Enforcement Agency (DEA) guys in their bulletproof vests and helmets, but that was about as extreme as it got. And even those suspects were not killers.

I thought to myself that I might not be the man for this particular job. Many years later, when I drive that stretch of the Long Island Expressway, I return to that thought. I also realized I had no choice in the matter. I was responsible for investigating all fraud and official misconduct at 295 VA facilities, including medical centers, cemeteries, and two hundred and fifty thousand employees. I ran agents like Tom Valery up and down the east coast. I could not remember any of them ever investigating a doctor killing a patient. This seemed like a case that might require me to involve the FBI—a thought that did not thrill me.

I was pleased that traffic was moving at a crawl; I was not eager to jump into these unknown waters. But I am not a guy who passes the buck. And there was no one to whom to pass the buck to. From the time I picked up line one, I owned this case, whatever the cost or reward.

I grew up in Brooklyn, both my parents were civil service workers and they pushed me in their direction. I attended Thomas Jefferson High School, a school with the reputation for a street-tough student body and a football team to prove it. The only jewelry I wore was my high school ring. The only decoration on the wall of my office was my diploma from Thomas Jefferson High School. On several occasions over my career, colleagues or suspects would notice the diploma and ask if I knew the school's legendary football coach Moe Finkelstein. I knew him and would say so.

They assumed I played football for Moe. I never said I did, but they would take a step back and think I was a tough guy with a tough background. I would notice a new level of respect from then on and I liked it.

In truth, I was aware my toughness came more from my mind than my body. After high school, I went to nearby Long Island University, where I also received my master's degree in political science. I could be like a dog with a bone but would rather outsmart opponents, be they embezzlers, drug dealers, or bureaucrats getting in my way. I was Columbo, not Dirty Harry.

As we approached Northport, I laid out a strategy. I thought I should have watched the television show the psychiatrist mentioned before we left the office. I wondered why nobody gave me a heads-up about it. Usually the press office in DC was on top of those things. Tom appeared to know all about it.

I understood I should not be so sure that we were on to a homicide case. So far, we were moving forward based solely on a panicky phone call from a psychiatrist I did not even know, and what was probably a lot of speculation from a television program.

If this did turn into something I knew I would have to prepare a thorough buttoned-up case so an Assistant US Attorney (AUSA) would be able to secure an indictment that would hold up in federal court. One AUSA once described me as "rock steady." That is what I needed to be now. My days of knocking down the doors of lowlifes who were stealing drugs from the VA medical center to sell on the street were far behind me. I never fired a shot in anger and hoped I never had to.

I knew I would have to call in the FBI if today's interview developed any real leads. They knew how to deal with a killer, if, indeed, we're dealing with one.

But in the meantime, this case was mine.

A detective relies on his experience. As special agent-in-charge, I knew my duty was to get to the bottom of the Swango story—even if the bottom was a dark place where I'd never ventured before and where the VA would not be happy about my shedding any light.

I shared my thoughts with Tom, who took a harder position. He didn't think the television report would have implicated Swango the way it did if the reporters behind it weren't sure.

He wasn't concerned about moving in against a possible killer who might be more aggressive about avoiding arrest than the bookkeeper we arrested last week for stealing petty cash to finance a sweet-sixteen for his daughter. Tom was a genuine tough guy, fearless and impatient with paperwork and forensic accountants. He wanted to do a murder case. We were both excited by the challenge.

At Northport, we met up with VA Police Chief Hank Shemitz, who was in charge of the uniformed forces there. Shemitz had done some preliminary work and shared that Swango was a psychiatric resident at nearby Stony Brook University Hospital. Under a routine agreement with the VA, Swango was doing a rotation at Northport. Shemitz said Swango appeared to be a skilled liar, a con man. When he applied for the job as a psychiatric resident, he never told the administrators anything about what the television show claimed—like the fact that he served time for poisoning fellow paramedics by putting ant killer in their donuts.

Shemitz said Swango admitted to having trouble with the law. He said he was in a bar with a number of paramedics with whom he worked; they ribbed him about being a doctor and getting his thrills riding around with them. He told Stony Brook that as an ex-Marine, he was not used to being ridiculed; he admitted losing his temper, starting a brawl and roughing up some of his colleagues. He said he served some time but was eventually exonerated by the governor of Virginia. He was so smooth that he was hired without a further background check.

Though Shemitz found it hard to believe they didn't do a formal background check, he told us that the university was having a difficult time filling certain job openings and they may have been eager to get a well-educated ex-Marine on their staff. Shemitz added, "When you meet this guy, you might understand how they were influenced by him."

I was stunned about the lack of any background check. It was inexcusable. I was embarrassed that the VA was now caught up in a possible fraud case because the suits at Stony Brook were taken in by a liar. Before joining the VA, I worked as an investigator for the Department of Defense doing background checks on people needing top-secret clearances. I had an uncanny ability to sniff out a liar. And I knew by experience, it rarely took much digging to uncover one. "This guy must be some operator," I thought.

Shemitz had spoken to the psychiatrist who called me because of the television show, which reported that Swango poisoned the paramedics and had a reputation for his patients dying unexpectedly. She was afraid that Swango might have committed crimes—even murder—at Northport. As Tom had told me back in the office, the program said Swango was nicknamed "Double O Swango, Licensed to Kill," at a hospital where he worked in Ohio, and he was asked to resign under suspicious circumstances. The television program alleged a trail of death followed wherever he went, including the suicide of his fiancée.

I was a little pissed at Tom for not calling me the night he had seen the show. It might have given me time to prepare a little better. Maybe I could have initiated the call to Northport and taken the lead instead of following up on Doctor Thomesen's call.

But here I was listening to these incredible stories about Swango. On the surface, it sounded like he committed fraud. That was in my ballpark, and easy to prove if Swango lied to the administrators. But murder! Where was the proof? That was a whole new ballgame.

The Northport medical center looked more like a college campus than a hospital. Surrounded by trees and lawns, there was a peaceful, healing atmosphere about the property. It even had a golf course.

Shemitz had arranged for a small room in the residents' dormitory for the sit-down with Swango. It was early fall and the tiny air conditioner was losing its battle against the midday sun. The three of us were crowded in the room, me in my blue pinstriped Brooks Brothers suit, which was as much a uniform as Shemitz's blue military-type outfit. We took the only two chairs. Tom removed his sport jacket and sat on the bed. The Glock on his hip was clearly visible. It was a technique he used to intimidate a suspect, even if the suspected crime was petty theft.

"So, do you think we have a killer on our hands?" I asked Shemitz as we settled in to wait.

"Who knows?" Shemitz answered. "This is new ground to me. I can't imagine a guy, whose friends call him "Doctor Death," could have gotten away with murder for so long."

I wondered the same thing. I never imagined I would find myself on the trail of a killer. "We've got to proceed very carefully," I said. "Clearly, he committed fraud when he lied to the Stony Brook admissions people, and we'll nail him for that. But murder? That remains to be seen."

Sitting and waiting for Swango, I thought back to those military candidates in their apartments or dorm rooms where the conditions were not always comfortable—not unlike the room we were in now.

Swango arrived right on time.

When he walked into the room, he looked like he had just come off the golf course. He was tanned, wearing a bright white and blue sweater, aviator sunglasses, full head of shiny hair—he radiated a movie star presence.

He nodded all around as I introduced the three of us and seeing no place to sit, took a spot on the bed next to Tom. It was just where I wanted him. I asked him if he was comfortable because I wanted him to think more about a cramp in his leg than what his next lie to me would be. He said he was fine. He appeared not to have a care in the world. He struck me as the kind of guy I would introduce to my daughter.

I thanked the doctor for joining us and started in on my usual banter to make the subject feel comfortable and among friends. I had done this thousands of times, like a singer performing his big hit at every show. Usually, I was focused on where I had to take the conversation next. But now my mind was going a mile a minute. I was actually a little nervous. I could not remember the last time I felt this way about engaging a suspect. I wished I had never heard about the possibility that Swango was a killer—and a serial killer at that. If this was just about fraud, I could have wrapped it up in five minutes.

But I am a control freak about investigations and that goes to my own composure as well. I stuck with my tried and true interrogation technique: I feigned disbelief at the allegations against the suspect. I wanted Swango to believe that I could not imagine he was capable of being guilty. I was the good cop. Tom would weigh in as the bad guy when and if it became necessary. Shemitz, in his dark blue uniform, was the reminder of the authority of the US government.

"Could this be you?" I asked the young doctor. "Is this television show correct? Did you poison fellow paramedics in Illinois? I find it hard to believe a man like you would have done this. Tell me the truth—let's clear it up." Tom recognized me in action. I knew he was enjoying a silent laugh knowing that my first question to my usual adversaries was more likely to be, "Did you possibly misappropriate some money from a patient's account?" Nothing about poison!

Tom, playing his role, stood up and leaned over the doctor. By now, his face was red from the heat, his shirt was sweat-stained, and the Glock looked like a Howitzer. "The show made it sound like you murdered patients. Where did they get that? Now's your time to get this cleared up before it gets out of control," Tom said, as he moved his right hand to the holster on his hip.

Tom then stepped away from the bed and took up position at the door. If Swango bolted, he was ready to stop him.

I leaned back in my chair, waited a beat or two, and then looked Swango in the eye. It was a clear signal I was waiting to hear the answer and I was sending the message: *You can deal with me or deal with my partner.*

Swango did not blink at the question. He completely maintained his composure. He shifted the dynamic and took charge. Not only was he a former Marine but he also came from a military family. He was totally self-assured. He looked right back into my eyes. "This is all gossip and bull-shit," he said. Turning toward Shemitz, he explained that he was framed. He said the paramedics he was convicted of poisoning hated him for his success, his genius as a doctor, and his good looks. He stood up and turned towards Tomas if to say, "*I'm not afraid of you.*" He pointed his finger at the agent and declared the governor of Virginia had restored all his civil rights after he served two and a half years of his five-year term. Then he slowly sat back down on the bed, refusing to be uncomfortable. I admit his performance had its effect. If he was lying, he clearly was an expert at it. Physically, he put out the message he was ready for anything, even Tom.

I was floored. I never expected such a performance. I looked across at Tom, who had a big smile on his face. He was engaged in battle and loved it.

I returned to Swango. "So, Doctor Swango, you are telling me that everything we have heard—all the gossip and the television show—is all nonsense? Just the product of envious colleagues?

"You never poisoned your colleagues' iced tea or brought them arsenic-laced donuts like the show reported?"

These questions bothered him and Swango's composure slipped a bit. His jaw stiffened and he pursed his lips. He was sweating now like the rest of us in the tight room. But he answered like a fighter who just got punched in the nose but keeps charging ahead. "You got that right, agent."

My composure did not slip. I stuck to my script and continued punching away.

"Of course, they were envious. Who wouldn't be? You seem to have everything going for you. Great education, good

17

looks, and you're probably a great doctor. It's easy to see why people would want to knock you down," I said.

I had heard denials like this before. Not necessarily from killers, but from embezzlers who were stealing VA money, mopes who stole the identities of true heroes in order to steal their benefits, or even from some physicians who faked reports in search of promotions. I knew there was always something they were hiding. Allegations like the television show made or like those I pursued in VA medical centers across the country never came from whole cloth. There was always an angle that weighed against the suspect. The challenge was to find it.

Valery was thinking the same thing: liar. He stole a glance at me and I nodded to him in return. We were on the same page. We were not about to swallow the story hook, line, and sinker, as the Stony Brook administration, to their disgrace, apparently had done.

At that moment, I was struck by thoughts that would haunt me for years to come: *If Swango is capable of poisoning his coworkers—paramedics, no less—would he go further? Could the poison have killed them? Could he control poison that effectively? How deranged is this guy with the movie star looks and doctor's brain? And how can he be stopped?*

I probed a little more. I wanted to move on from the television show. What was Swango's life like? I asked what schools he attended, and where he served in the Marines. Was he married? Did he have a girlfriend? I asked the kinds of questions I would ask candidates for a top-secret clearance.

I followed my tried-and-true line of questioning about where he liked to go on vacation, but before he could answer, I doubled back to the television show. I asked him why the television show would present such an incriminating report. I asked if he planned on suing the show. "After all," I said, "they may have damaged your reputation beyond repair. It may be impossible for you to get a good position anywhere. You're obviously a talented guy; you're a Marine veteran. Surely, you're not going to take this lying down," I said, trying to bait him into some kind of admission.

He stuck to his story, determined to always point to a conspiracy against a brilliant, handsome doctor that he was tired of fighting. And then he slipped a little again. "I wouldn't waste my time fighting this," he said. It was a common answer from those who have run out of rational lies and were not ready to tell the truth. But unlike suspects I had arrested over the years, instead of giving in and facing the inevitable, he quickly regained his swagger. He had the balls to scold me: "This questioning is an affront to my talents as a doctor and the good work I do."

I realized I would not get anything more out of Swango at this interview, but I did not want to leave without uncovering something that was not in the television show—something that Swango could not deny.

I made a gambit that I had used many times before: I asked if we could search his room. If I was dealing with an embezzler, I might be looking for money or a set of bogus account books. For an ID thief, I might hope to find forged or stolen identification cards. I had no idea what I might find in the room of a serial killer, but I did not want to leave empty-handed, with no advancement of what the television show reported. I was afraid to leave any stone unturned. I wanted to look at the private life of a man who might be a homicidal maniac.

For the first time since our session began, Swango's face betrayed him. The request to see his room clearly caught him off guard. He did not answer immediately. Then he balked at the request. He vehemently refused. He stood as Tom, Shemitz, and then I filed out of the room, and angrily declared we would need a court order to search his room. I kept walking away, stopping Tom from going back in to give the doctor some shit. If I needed any incentive to keep pursuing this guy, I now had it. I knew in my gut that Swango was hiding something that would make things worse for him. I no longer thought I would like my daughter to meet him.

In the hallway outside the room, the three of us agreed that Swango was not telling us the whole story. Was he a killer? He offered no evidence of that. It was outside our realm of experience, but we needed to determine what was true.

The first step was to visit nearby Stony Brook University Hospital to find out if Swango really did lie on his admission papers.

"If we determine he lied, we at least have a fraud case against him," I said. "We have a clear direction to follow. Anything else is probably going to take a lot more digging and maybe some resources we don't presently have."

The admission officials at Stony Brook assured me they were moving quickly to complete the background check, which should have been done four months before they hired Swango. Everyone was talking about the television show, and while I now realized how Swango's charm and confidence could have fooled the entrance committee at Stony Brook, I was aghast that no one even thought to look past his initial application and interview to check him out. I was embarrassed the VA might have shared responsibility for enabling a monster to treat patients at Northport. As the administrator fumbled through his excuses, I made a mental list of people who had to be contacted about just who Swango was, breaking it down into tasks for Tom and myself.

Before leaving Northport, I used the phone in Shemitz's office to call Loretta Lynch, Chief Assistant U.S. Attorney in the Eastern District of New York. Based in Brooklyn, the Eastern District had jurisdiction over Suffolk County, where Northport is located. VA medical centers are considered federal reservations and legal jurisdiction falls to federal authorities, similar to crimes on a military base.

Lynch, the future attorney general in the Obama administration, listened carefully to my recounting of the television program. Once again, I kicked myself for not taking the time to watch it before we left the office. I recounted the call from the psychiatrist and the meeting with Swango, which hadn't gone as well as I would have liked. I guess I was hoping he would have confessed and come back to New York in handcuffs. I told Lynch I would really like to get into the doctor's room.

I pleaded with every bone in my special agent body to get in there, but Lynch was a smart cookie and not easy to manipulate. She said I had no probable cause, as there was no evidence the doctor had committed any crimes at the Northport facility. A television show's speculation did not represent proper evidence. No probable cause equaled no warrant and no amount of my pleading could budge her. Nor should it have.

I was disappointed but not surprised. I knew the rules and I knew Lynch played by them. I told Tom we could expect a call from the FBI that set off a minute or two of cursing under his breath—about the *Famous But Incompetent* blowhards and big-foot amateurs, which were his longtime favorite objects of derision. I preferred to call them the *Federal Bureau of Arrogance*. We both knew Lynch was too good a prosecutor to ignore what I had told her. Even though there was no immediate action she could approve, I knew she would share the Swango lead with the Bureau and would initiate an investigation by them. That was her job. She could not let suspicions about a possible criminal go uninvestigated. But it was not just about covering her ass. Lynch understood my instincts were usually right on and I could probably use the support of the feds.

I always found working with them to be difficult. But deep down, I knew I would need their resources to investigate a crime that might require numerous interviews in a few states and, perhaps,, scientific research before anything could be uncovered. It was going to be aggravation because they always big-footed any agency that wasn't theirs. But, if Lynch could get a warrant signed by a federal judge that would allow me to search Swango's room, it was worth the potential aggravation it might bring. Tom didn't agree. He hated the FBI. "Fuck'em," he told me. "Let's just do what we have to do and bring this guy in and let Lynch work it out." Tom knew it was not my style. Frankly. I enjoyed his ranting from time to time. It was a way of blowing off steam and worked for me by osmosis.

Driving back to Manhattan, we shared our amazement about the events of the past few hours. We were convinced Swango was a liar but not certain he was a killer. I told Tom to make Swango his number one priority. I told him to hit the phones, contacts, and reach out anywhere Swango had ever lived and worked. I wanted him to find out what he could about this strange person who needed to be stopped in his tracks. I assured him I would handle the brass, try to cut red tape and soothe the hurt feelings among hospital employees our investigation was sure to cause. More significantly, I would line up the type of experts we would need to prove Swango was a killer.

That evening over dinner, I told my wife, Eileen, about the events of the day. She had read a newspaper account of the television program. It was the talk of our block in Massapequa, Long Island, which was not very far from Northport. Many of our neighbors had relatives, especially World War II Vietnam vets, who were treated at Northport. Eileen thought it was scary to think of a serial killer on the loose in a hospital. She urged me to be careful, not so much for my personal safety but for my professional standing. She understood I was in uncharted territory and already had a case to make against the administrators at Northport for not doing their own background check on Swango. She realized I would be stepping on many toes if this turned into a worst-case scenario. The VA might not be so happy with me if I ended up proving one of its doctors was a serial killer. It could dead-end my career. But she understood I had no choice but to carry on.

Two days later, Shemitz called me to report Swango had been fired at Stony Brook and had moved out of his dormitory room to parts unknown. No charges were filed alleging he committed any crimes at Northport. I was incredulous and asked the chief, "Do they realize they might have let a killer escape justice?" He had no good answer. It wasn't his doing so I held my tongue. But as soon as I hung up on Shemitz, I called Tom into my office.

"Can you imagine they let Swango take off? Shemitz has no idea where he has gone. I can't believe no one was watching him," I told my right-hand man.

Tom was sympathetic towards the chief. "The Stony Brook brass must have been breathing down the necks of the Northport people," he said. "You know, if there is something really fugazy here, they don't want it out; they want it under the rug. They don't want us near Swango."

I knew Tom was correct. Stony Brook's error in hiring him without a thorough background check was a mistake of enormous magnitude—especially now that Swango had been partially exposed. I know they had no grounds to hold him, but undoubtedly, they made matters worse by letting him slip away. Again, I cursed the fact I could not get into Swango's room. Maybe, I thought for the thousandth time, I would have found something there that would have allowed me to detain the bastard. Well, I couldn't keep crying over spilled milk. I had to figure out what I could do now. I swore Doctor Michael Swango had not seen the last of me.

Thankfully, old, reliable Tom had been busy since we left Northport. He was making calls delving into Swango's mysterious past. He confirmed with law enforcement in Illinois that Swango served two and a half years in prison for poisoning paramedics.

Tom spoke to Swango's fellow medical students and the mother of a former fiancée of Swango, whose daughter had committed suicide. She blamed Swango for driving her daughter insane. Tom's preliminary work convinced us both that the man we interviewed in the sweatbox at Northport was a killer, and we were hot on his trail. Except we did not know where he was.

About a week after our visit to Northport, I received the call I had been expecting. A meeting was arranged between my office and the New York office of the FBI.

At the confab, I suggested the US Attorney, the FBI, and my team pursue a fraud investigation of Swango for misrepresenting his background while digging deeper into the possibility that he had committed murder. "We need to buy the time to make this a homicide case," I said.

The FBI supervisor patiently allowed me to lay out my strategy. He smiled and nodded his head in agreement. He took some notes. He said "good idea" a couple of times. Then he shot it all to hell.

He said he did not care about pursuing fraud. He declared the FBI would take over the entire investigation and look at the potential murder case. He would not work jointly with us. He said the very fact that Swango was allowed to practice at Northport in the first place was an example of VA incompetence that I, as special agent in charge, should have caught. The FBI would pursue a murder investigation even though there was not a shred of evidence anyone had been harmed. It was contradictory and typical bigfooting by the *Famous But Incompetent* and it was humiliating for me to sit in the big conference room surrounded by senior agents and listen to it. But looking on the bright side, it did at least indicate that they were afraid to totally dismiss what my instinct was telling me. They believed me but didn't want me around. It was similar to turning down financial help from your in-laws because you don't want them to visit.

I was seething when Tom and I, tails between our legs, returned to our office a few blocks north of FBI headquarters. Once again, the Bureau would bigfoot another agency's case. This was a complaint shared by law enforcement officers from local traffic cops to senior investigators in the DEA. When the FBI got involved, it became their case. They got all the glory—but if things went south, you took the blame.

I had a bad FBI taste in my mouth since the 1970s, when the federal government established a separate Office of Inspector General for all major agencies. The Bureau argued back then that separate agencies should not have their own investigative staffs and opposed their having law enforcement authority. In my early days as a VA OIG investigator, I had to be sworn in as a Special Deputy US Marshal when pursuing a case. It was a hindrance and humiliating. Finally, Congress resisted the FBI's lobbying and granted law enforcement powers to the OIGs against the wishes of the Bureau. It was a sore point, which still stuck in the craw of agents of my generation. It was all about the FBI seeing itself as the premier cops of the nation and wanting to keep it that way no matter how many bureaucratic obstacles and blown cases were caused by their attitude.

By the time we got back to our office, a call had come in that the Bureau wanted all the medical records of Swango's patients and copies of anything else pertaining to the investigation. Of course, because the allegations against Swango involved a VA medical center, we had control of the records. I informed them they would need a court order to get those records.

They obviously did not like my answer because that same day I received a call from the brand-new US Attorney for the Eastern District of New York, the big dog himself, Zachary Carter. In a very straightforward conversation, he threatened me with obstruction of justice if I did not release those records to his office.

With great patience, with no hint of sarcasm, I explained that the records were property of the Veterans Administration. They were not mine to release. It would be interesting if his criminal division prosecuted me for obstruction of justice for not releasing the records, while his civil division defended me for following the law.

Once again, rather than ordering a joint investigation, which would have made the records and all my resources available to the FBI, they went to court and got the court orders. For the moment, the *Federal Bureau of Arrogance* triumphed.

But I knew how to survive this inter-agency competition. Deep down inside, I did not believe the FBI had taken me seriously. If they had, they would have accepted my strategy and moved forward with developing the fraud case first. But they didn't, and so now, I did not want to let go of Swango.

"Let the VA turn the records over, but make copies for us," I told Tom, "because we're going to stay on his trail. Serial killers don't take vacations. Let me know anything you dig up about him. I'm going to learn all I can about doctors who kill. There must be books out there about sensational cases. Maybe some of the old-timers remember a case or two. I need to find out how to prove our case when we're ready to bring it to court. When Swango pops up again, we are going to nail him for murder."

I might have been a white-collar crime investigator in the morning but on the way home that night, I knew I was now a homicide detective. I got a charge out of thinking about it. This was the beginning of an adventure and I was excited to get rolling.

CHAPTER 3

Buicks and Bad Guys

"If we do not maintain justice, justice will not maintain us."

—SIR FRANCIS BACON

So, we got the boot from the FBI. I can't say that surprised me, but I was surprising myself with how much it was bothering me. I offered them a good plan. Pick up Swango on the charge he lied to Stony Brook and hold him while I dug deeper into his suspicious past. The blind arrogance of the Bureau rejected it.

It was rare for me to take my work home but that night at dinner, I passed on my frustration to Eileen, who patiently listened and agreed with me that they were being jerks. After dinner, we watched TV, but I was restless and knew I would not sleep that night.

I went off to the two-car garage where my prize possession, a 1938 Buick Limited Model 91, sat waiting for my attention. Classic cars were my passion, and this was a real beauty. If anything could take my mind off Doctor Michael Swango, an hour or two of polishing old Betsy would do it.

I would buy a classic that needed mostly cosmetic work and then fuss over it like a newborn baby. This particular model reminded me of World War II days. It was one of the last prewar models. It was also the last model that Buick used actual wood for in production. To me, it evoked movie images of war era leaders arriving for meetings and GIs parking them in their driveways after the war.

I have great affection for the World War II veterans. My father was one as were so many of the fathers and uncles who lived in my neighborhood when I was growing up. They wore Army surplus "Ike" jackets and pants and drove cars like the 1938 Buick. They deserved to be honored. They deserved to be remembered.

My work was investigating crimes against veterans and I was proud to be their guardian. I knew, as I put my can of Simonize away, I would never be comfortable with the idea that a doctor was preying on these guys on my watch while I was being prevented from doing something about it. Well, I was not going to let that happen.

I was too anxious to sleep well. Conflicting thoughts kept me awake. I wanted to get Swango but I admit I questioned my ability to do it. By five o'clock in the morning, I was on the Long Island Railroad headed for Manhattan.

Forty-five minutes later, regular coffee in hand, I was walking into our office on Seventh Avenue and 24thTwenty-Fourth Street, across the street from the Fashion Institute of Technology—where artists and designers learned how to conquer the world of fashion.

My office was on the sixteenth floor of a building that housed several government agencies. It was a seventeen-story building, but the last elevator stop was the sixteenth floor. The next floor was rumored to be secret offices of the CIA. I don't know how they got there, maybe up a concealed staircase in the rear of the building, but I totally believed the rumors.

Tom greeted me when I walked in. He was the only person there. Most of the staff arrived around nine o'clock. He smelled a little like burnt wood, which told me he was up late fighting a fire, and decided to come straight in to work. On his desk was a brand-new manila folder marked "Swango."

"Good," I thought; we were on the same page.

I settled in behind my desk that I took pride in keeping neat, and asked Tom if he thought Swango could really be a killer and how would we ever prove it.

How does he kill patients, and no one notices? We would need to ask Doctor Thomesen at Northport which patients she thinks Swango killed. If there were complaints of that nature, it would have come to my desk unless someone was covering them up. I told him to speak to the television producers who did the sensational program. Why did they think Swango was a killer?

Tom said he definitely made Swango out as a smooth-talking con man. He had the aura of confidence we had seen many times in embezzlers and ID thieves. But they were not killers.

What could Swango use for a weapon?

"Maybe he smothered them with a pillow, cut off their IV, or disconnected their oxygen. Maybe he gave them an injection of poison. If they were seriously ill, no one would question it," Tom said.

That was all possible. But wouldn't someone notice? How brazen he must be doing that on a busy ward!

"Hey boss, you've been to a hospital. When the doctor pulls that curtain around the bed, no one knows what's going on behind it besides him. You don't even know what he's doing to you. It's not a bad place to commit a murder and get away with it." My partner's words sent a chill down my spine. Suddenly, I had a vivid memory of being in the hospital when I was fourteen years old. I hadn't thought of that in years.

My appendix burst and I was rushed to Brookdale Hospital, the "go-to" emergency room for my Brooklyn neighborhood. Nurses were fussing over me and every once in a while, a young doctor would appear, put his stethoscope to my chest, and feel my side. My distraught mother came up to my gurney and gave me the news I would need an operation to remove my appendix. She tried to calm me by saying it was a common operation and everything would turn out well.

I was happy to believe her. But I was scared and tried not to cry from the pain, when my attention completely shifted to a raucous scene developing before my eyes.

I saw the police rolling in two Hispanic men who were neighbors of mine in the housing project in which we lived. They had both been stabbed in some kind of fight. They were screaming curses at the medics trying to help them while struggling to get off their gurneys and out the door. I was chilled as one screamed, "You're killing me, I can't take it anymore, won't someone please help me?"

The cops had their hands full restraining them. Then their family members came charging into the ER. I recognized many of them. They were yelling at everyone, even the medical staff working furiously to save the lives of the two men. It was bedlam. Then silence!

One of the men on the gurney died! The medics stopped working. They slowly withdrew from him. They looked at each other, one of them nodded, and another pulled a sheet over the man's face. I was terrified. I had never even been in a hospital before much less five feet from a dead man.

The second stabbing victim now, instead of calming down, jumped off the gurney and tried to leave. It took two cops and a burly nurse's aide to get him back on the gurney. This time they strapped him down. His body was shaking uncontrollably, and they rolled him a couple of feet and pulled a curtain around him.

Afraid as I was for my life, I was fixated on what was going on behind the curtain. I could not see anything, but I could hear the staff arguing about the treatment they gave the man who died. One was saying they could have done more. Another was arguing they did all they could, and it was hopeless to save him.

Right there in the center of the ER, a doctor broke the news to the dead man's family. He said they did all they could. They did not take the news well. They were overcome by grief. They asked no questions about the treatment.

As a fourteen-year-old, I remember asking myself if the doctors in the Brookdale ER lied to the family. Could the man have been saved?

Now, sitting across from Tom, as I think of veterans dying in Northport, who is asking questions? Has anyone checked on Swango's patients, the ones who died, that is? Who could his loved ones ask?

I recovered well from my appendix surgery and thirty years later, I am remembering the questions I asked myself then. Well, now, maybe I can get some answers.

Tom noticed I was distracted,,but snapped me back.

"So boss, what the fuck are we going to do here?" he asked.

I mulled it over for a minute or two and then I answered. We would have to map out a strategy to pursue this case without running into an FBI roadblock. We knew we couldn't clear our desks of our ongoing investigations, but maybe we could carve out time for Swango.

Tom said he was carrying a light load at the time and would be on the phones immediately.

"Well, I've got to finally pull the trigger on that Greenberg case," I said. "I've been hesitating because I know the guy, but I'm going to get a postal inspector to back me up and head out to Great Neck for the collar."

"Is Alvin Greenberg the guy who works in this building?" Tom asked.

"Yeah! I see him in the lobby and elevator all the time. He's a lawyer whose job is to advocate for veterans who need help. But he's been fucking over an African American veteran named Fred Green. Fred was a soldier in the Red Ball Express, one of the truckers who saved Patton's army when it ran out of fuel during the Battle of the Bulge. My father was a tank trooper for Patton. He told me the story many times about how they waited helplessly in the frozen woodlands for fuel as the Germans made their last-ditch effort to stop the Allies.

"When those trucks, with the big red balls painted on the doors, came barreling down the road, they knew they were saved and the Germans were toast."

A few months before, I received a call from a social worker at a shelter in the Bronx. Fred had been taken there by firefighters, who found him alone in a dilapidated, vermin-infested apartment with no running water and only a kerosene heater for warmth that had caught fire. In the debris was a photo of Fred as a strapping young GI. The firefighters took it with them, along with some official-looking papers, when they brought Fred to the adult care facility. There was nothing else worth taking.

Fred was not able to tell the social worker much about himself. But I was able to track his records. I discovered he came home ill from Europe and was diagnosed as *not competent* to handle his own affairs. His brother was declared his legal guardian, took care of him for about fifty years, and managed to put away forty-five thousand dollars for Fred before he passed away.

When I went to visit Fred, he could not make much sense of anything except he believed he did not have any money. He showed me a letter from the VA dated a year after his brother died that declared him *competent* to handle his own affairs.

I asked him what he did with the money his brother helped him save.

Fred was barely coherent, but he mumbled, "My attorney, Greenberg, has my money. He takes care of me." Greenberg signed the *competency* letter.

What a disgrace! This helpless war hero was malnourished, dirty, and suffering from several chronic diseases. He was left to die in a firetrap.

Fred was a sweet guy, the kind of guy you want to hug. To think he was taken so advantage of made my blood boil. He may have saved my father's life. I needed to get justice for him.

With the help of postal inspectors and a VA forensic accountant from our staff, we figured Greenberg manipulated records and his own interviews with Fred to have the veteran declared competent so that he could gain control over his funds—*and* the dead brother's estate. Through a complicated web of financial transactions, Greenberg transferred Fred's money to his personal accounts, then used it with money he stole from other veterans; he financed a swanky Long Island bachelor pad for himself, and a lavish wedding and house in Florida for his daughter.

I could only wonder why no one in the House Committee on Veterans Affairs was bothered by the fact the veteran was *incompetent* for thirty-five years and then all of a sudden was *competent*. Someone should have flagged that to the Inspector General's Office, my office, before those firefighters found Fred in desperate straits.

And it turned out Greenberg did not limit his felony to Fred. We discovered he eventually embezzled more than one hundred and twenty-five thousand dollars from other veterans.

Two days after deciding to clear my desk so I could concentrate on Swango, a postal inspector and I went out to Greenberg's mini-mansion in Great Neck, Long Island, and knocked on the door. Greenberg, who considered himself a ladies' man, was dressed in light blue slacks, with a cashmere V-neck sweater, loafers, and sunglasses. He looked like he was ready for a date on the French Riviera.

When he saw me, though, he knew he was heading for a date with a judge. I identified myself and placed him under arrest.

"Don't I know you?" he said. "You're behind this, aren't you? Don't we work in the same building?"

"Not anymore," I replied.

At his sentencing a year later, Judge Kenneth Conboy said to Greenberg, "This is a monstrous crime you are convicted of," and sentenced him to three years in jail and ordered full restitution to the veterans. After serving his sentence, Greenberg was ordered to perform community service at a VA medical center for the mentally ill.

Over the next few weeks, I dispatched a few more typical cases, believing we would learn any day that Swango had
resurfaced somewhere. But after a while, I began to realize it
might take a little longer to nail the elusive con man.

Thankfully, Tom was putting the time to good use. He
was aggressively building a file on Swango. A file that eventually read like the notebook of Hannibal Lecter.

CHAPTER 4

The Monster Returns

"Destroy the seed of evil, or it will grow up to your ruin."

—AESOP

Originally, I thought it might take a few months to track down a smooth con artist like Swango. I was certain he would try to land another medical job and turn up on the FBI's radar before too long. Well, I was wrong. Months passed with no word on Swango. I sometimes thought it was possible the Bureau had picked him up and dealt with him on the fraud charge without even letting me know. I would not put that past them; realistically, I thought we would hear something—at least from the grapevine—if that happened.

Don't get me wrong! I wasn't discouraged. I was used to investigations taking a long time. And Valery was doing a good job updating me. For each day that went by, I became more and more determined to nail the guy.

I finally watched the television program that set off the alarms at Northport, over and over again, and took notes.

Tom stayed in close contact with Charlene Thomesen, the forensic psychiatrist who called me the morning I went out to Northport. From records and anecdotal evidence she was able to turn up, the doctor was able to build a psychological profile of Swango. And I continued my "medical" research and reached out to some retired investigators to ask if they ever encountered the possibility of a killer on the loose in one of our hospitals.

We now established a dossier going back as far as we could into Swango's past. Swango's father, a career Army officer, returned from Vietnam with an alcohol problem. He often talked to his three children—Michael was the middle child—about his war experiences, and especially the killings in which he participated. By all accounts it was a dysfunctional household, and when Swango was still a young boy, his parents divorced. He grew up in Quincy, Illinois, along the banks of the Mississippi River at the state's western border. Despite the upsetting home life, his activities included playing the clarinet in the band at Quincy Catholic Boys High School, and he graduated valedictorian from there in 1972.

After high school, Swango served four years in the Marines without seeing action overseas. In the Marines, I learned, Swango became fanatic about his physical condition and became a lifelong devotee of push-ups and jogging as a means of self-discipline. One of his medical school professors told me that if Swango was criticized over an even minor mistake, he would drop to the floor and perform fifty or so push-ups as a form of self-punishment. The other students would cheer him on.

Swango received an honorable discharge and enrolled in Quincy College in Illinois where he excelled in chemistry, graduated *summa cum laude* and received the American Chemical Society Award.

It sounded pretty good so far. But at Southern Illinois University School of Medicine (SIU), where he next enrolled, we found from interviews with officials there that his classmates noted some unusual behavior. It unsettled enough of his fellow medical students for them to bring it to the attention of supervisors. They said he was fascinated with dying patients. He hovered over their bedsides, studied their charts, and asked questions about what kind of pain they were in and how they were bearing it. And while he was considered a brilliant student, with the potential of being a great doctor, no one got the impression he was searching for ways to help those desperate patients. It appeared that what he enjoyed most was being close to their suffering.

His colleagues also thought he was lazy. They found it odd that he preferred working with an ambulance crew to studying. And a look back at records showed that an unusual number of patients with whom he came into contact ended up "coding"—that is, experiencing unexpected life-threatening episodes. Five of them had died.

It was at SIU that students began referring to him as "Double O Swango, Licensed to Kill," for his cavalier attitude toward death and mishandling of cadavers. He hit a major bump in the road at SIU when fellow students complained to the disciplinary committee that he had been faking reports on ob-gyn patients, which indicated he had been doing checkups on them. He narrowly missed being expelled; when one member of the committee voted to give him a second chance, he was forced to repeat his ob-gyn rotation, which caused him to graduate a year later than planned.

By now, he had gained a strange, dark reputation and a poor evaluation from SIU. Nevertheless, he obtained a surgical internship at Ohio State University (OSU) Medical Center in 1983 and then a residency in neurosurgery. I thought this was incredible! When I learned this, I thought Stony Brook wasn't the first place taken in by his con-man act.

I always had great respect for nurses. I interviewed dozens of them over the years as part of all kinds of investigations, from staff stealing drugs and selling them on the street, to doctors faking reports. I always found them forthright, always putting their patients first. I knew nurses would be essential to our efforts as we built our case against Swango.

At OSU, it was the nurses who complained that healthy patients were mysteriously dying with unexpected frequency whenever Swango was the intern on their floor. One nurse caught him injecting something into a patient who later became ill. The nurses reported their concerns, but the administration conducted a very superficial investigation and then dismissed the complaining nurses as paranoid. This was a pattern I would see often over the next few years. Hospital brass never wanted to hear bad news about their doctors. Too often, they were willing to cover up in order to save face.

What I eventually learned from studying OSU reports reads like the script from a horror movie. Gossip about Swango began in earnest while he was assigned to Rhodes Hall. In response, he was transferred to neighboring Doan Hall. On February 19, 1984, shortly after his transfer, Charlotte Warner, seventy-two years old, was found dead in her room. Only hours earlier, her doctor had told her she was doing well after a recent surgery, well enough to go home in a day. Something—someone—had caused her blood to clot in several organs. The same day, Evelyn Pereney began bleeding profusely from body orifices, even through her eyes, after being examined by Swango. The resident physician had no explanation for the hemorrhaging.

The following day, a twenty-two-year-old woman, recovering from a simple intestinal operation, rolled up her sleeve to permit Swango to give her a shot, as he later claimed, to increase her blood pressure. Swango pulled the curtain around him and the patient and asked the woman's mother to leave the room. The mother did not understand why the doctor wanted to shoo her from the room, but after a brief argument, she relented. A few minutes later, Swango confronted the woman with an attitude that seemed almost victorious. "She's dead now," Swango smirked. "You can go look at her."

Within a year, seven patients Swango had cared for as an OSU resident unexpectedly died. Five died shortly after Swango pulled the curtain around their bed for a private examination. When he left the room of a sixth patient, she immediately turned blue and stopped breathing. She survived and later told staff that Swango had put something in her IV just prior to her attack.

The seventh patient appeared to be recovering well from surgery but shortly after Swango visited her bedside during his rounds, she began to bleed from her nose and eyes and suffer total organ failure. Emergency treatment saved her, but it was later determined that her blood had failed to clot, a common reaction to poisoning.

When she recovered, she reported Swango injected something into her IV.

Around this time one of the strangest incidents in Swango's résumé of the bizarre occurred. Nineteen-year-old Cynthia McGee, who was attending the University of Illinois on a gymnastic scholarship, was run down by a speeding car while walking near the campus.

According to records we were able to examine from Ohio State University Medical Center and the investigation that followed, Cynthia was grievously injured. But she was otherwise healthy and possessed the strength and will of a world-class athlete. So, from the beginning, all signs indicated she would pull through.

Two months after the incident, the records indicated doctors thought she would benefit from being closer to her family, and she was in good enough health to be moved to a hospital closer to her home. She was transferred to the Ohio State University Medical Center in Columbus, where "Double O Swango" was working as a resident. It was Cynthia's misfortune that Swango was one of the doctors assigned to help her complete her recovery.

Days after Swango began caring for her, the strong young gymnast died suddenly. Swango was the last doctor to pull the curtain around her bedside in order to treat her. The next nurse to check on her found her dead. The news sent shock waves through the hospital.

Staffers were confounded by Cynthia's unexpected demise and raised questions with the hospital administration. The hospital conducted an internal investigation. Nurses demanded an outside law enforcement agency be called in, and when the hospital took its time, they complained to the local prosecutor, who launched an independent investigation.

Tom reached one of the assistant prosecutors who looked into the death of Cynthia McGee. The prosecutor's lawmen noted in their reports that they were blocked by the hospital administration at every turn, despite the fact that everywhere Swango went, "code blues and deaths by respiratory failure increased."

"Wherever Swango went, death was sure to follow," one prosecutor told Valery.

Eventually they exhumed five bodies in Ohio, but their evidence proved inconclusive and Swango escaped the law. After reading the prosecutor's extensive files, I no longer wondered whether I was pursuing a killer. I was convinced of it.

I couldn't believe my eyes when I read a notation in the OSU Medical Center file regarding a patient who complained about Swango and the IV she received. The notation, which would be permanently a part of her medical files, indicated that she was suffering from psychiatric problems due to her insistence that a doctor had tried to kill her.

The Cynthia McGee incident was shocking. The lawyer for the driver of the car that hit her told the media "She was making a "storybook recovery. Two or three days later, she was dead. We were sitting back here saying, 'what happened?' We knew something was wrong, but we couldn't prove it."

Scott Bone, seventeen, the driver of the car that hit McGee, was convicted of reckless homicide in her death and sentenced to thirty months of probation, one thousand hours of community service, and revocation of his license.

Reading the file was like reading the *Tales from the Crypt* comic books of my childhood. In those stories people died from the strangest, most unexpected terrors. Mad professors and deranged monsters found ways to torture and kill them, not brilliant young doctors who had sworn the Hippocratic Oath.

Fellow medical students saw Swango as a torturer. One day in June 1984, towards the end of his residency, Swango offered to buy take-out chicken for a group of physician coworkers. Tom learned that all the doctors who ate the chicken quickly began vomiting and developed diarrhea. All suspected Swango of "doctoring" the chicken, but nothing could be proven. Once again, he skated free because he apparently knew how to cover his crimes. Perhaps he used a substance that was not traceable in the bloodstream. Or perhaps, he thought no one even suspected something like that.

It was the last straw for Swango's colleagues and they quietly pressured OSU to cut them loose from what they saw as a killing machine. The University revoked its offer of a residency when Swango's internship ended. Incredibly, OSU gave Swango a glowing recommendation that allowed him to get his medical license. He was no longer a student but a full-fledged doctor—only now with a license to practice. He was free to find another killing ground.

CHAPTER 5

One of the Guys

"True friends stab you in the front."

—OSCAR WILDE

From Ohio, Swango returned to his hometown of Quincy, Illinois, two hours north of St. Louis. There, rather than try to land a job as a physician, he told people he was burned out by the demands of being a doctor and he signed on to the Adams County Ambulance Services as a medical technician.

Coworkers thought it was a little odd that a doctor, who could be making more money and enjoying the prestige of working at a major hospital, had instead chose to ride around in an ambulance. At all hours of the day and night, he gave advanced first aid to mostly vehicle accident and heart attack victims.

I spoke to some Quincy paramedics on the phone.

They clearly remembered Swango. Some had spoken with the television reporters and their stories became a part of the show. They said he had great interest in their accounts of serious accidents and crimes to which they responded. He

45

seemed obsessed with the news of a mass shooting in a fast-food restaurant.

Swango made a habit of bringing donuts and other fast food into the paramedics' headquarters, as a way of endearing himself to the rest of the first responders. He desperately wanted them to consider him just "one of the guys."

One day as four of the crew, but not Swango, sat around shooting the breeze at a small dining table in the room where they awaited response calls, they dug into a box of Swango's donuts with their coffee. Within minutes, they all began to feel queasy and experience some pain in their stomachs. One was forced to run to the men's room, where he became violently ill. He told investigators he thought he might be dying as he vomited worse than he had ever done in his life. He was sweating and dizzy as he made his way to a sleeping area used by paramedics on overnight shifts. After an hour or two, he recovered well enough to go home for rest.

That evening. Swango called the sick paramedic to ask him how he felt. He wanted to hear all the details about the vomiting, pain, and fear he was dying. The stricken man thought the call was strange, but thought it was prompted by Swango's background as a doctor.

"At first, I thought it was kind of him to check up on me. Maybe, I was thinking, he felt responsible because he brought the donuts in. But then he started to ask me for details of how I felt.

"He asked me how bad the pain was, how long it lasted. He wanted to know if I had spasms. Was I sweating? He asked me if I thought I was dying."

"After a few minutes, he was creeping me out. He was definitely enjoying hearing about my pain. I thought he was disappointed that I didn't die."

The others were not so badly affected; when they heard about the telephone call, they all realized something was wrong and suspected Swango of "doctoring" the donuts. They all agreed to keep a close eye on the doctor who preferred to work on an ambulance crew.

A few weeks later, some of the same group agreed they had to get to the bottom of their suspicions about their strange colleague. They brewed a pitcher of iced tea and left it on the coffee room table when they responded to a call without Swango.

When they returned from the call, instead of drinking the iced tea, they took it to a local laboratory and asked for it to be checked for any ingredients that did not belong in it. The lab report indicated it was packed with arsenic.

Back at headquarters, they searched through Swango's duffel bag, where they found a container of ant killer. The main ingredient of that particular ant killer was arsenic.

They took their suspicions and evidence to the Quincy police, who were convinced there was something to the complaints; The amateur detective work done by the paramedics helped them to obtain warrants to search Swango's home.

What they found there put any doubts they might have had about the suspect to rest. Swango had created a laboratory in his kitchen where he was clearly experimenting with poisons. He had dozens of chemicals on hand. He kept notes on index cards of the properties of different substances that could be used to make poisons, and on other cards, he created recipes for deadly concoctions. His library contained chemistry textbooks and books about death and the joy of killing.

"He killed for fun. He enjoyed watching people suffer," an investigator told me.

Faced with the Quincy city police's ever-mounting evidence of his crime, and the desire to get this sordid affair behind them, Swango was offered a fairly lenient plea deal.

On August 23, 1985, Swango was convicted of aggravated battery for poisoning the paramedics and sentenced to five years in prison. The sentencing judge had specific orders for the corrections department: Swango must not be allowed to work in the kitchen and must not be near preparation of any food for inmates or staff.

The case got a ton of publicity and it was especially noted back at OSU. Now, the OSU authorities conducted a serious internal investigation, including exhuming bodies of patients that unexpectedly died. They quickly determined they should have called in local law enforcement a year ago when so many of their trusted nurses, students, and a patient showed the courage to complain about Swango. Franklin County, Ohio prosecutors in Ohio stood by their previous decision proclaiming they did not have enough evidence to move forward with criminal cases.

But now information was flowing more freely. People were talking. I needed another agent on board. I took great pride in mentoring young agents, so I assigned Samantha Lockery, who had just transferred up from Washington, where she worked as an investigative assistant, to work with Tom. He was happy to have her aboard and as he had done with other young agents, he became like a father figure to her.

And now we were hot on the trail of Swango, or at least his history. The police investigation and subsequent trial had created a public record, which steered us to colleagues, victims, their families, and law enforcement personnel—from police officers to prosecutors and defense attorneys—we could reach out to for our own investigation.

Journalists who covered the trial were also helpful. The great television reporter John Stossel interviewed Swango for the program *20/20* at the Centralia Correctional Center in Illinois, where Swango was serving his five years.

Swango was his usual brazen self. He denied doing anything of which he was accused. He said the media concocted the story. He declared his innocence.

Stossel told him the public feared his release from jail. They didn't want him back on the streets, much less practicing medicine. Swango looked pained by the question and answered, "There's no reason for anyone to be scared. None whatsoever."

But what was starting to scare me was the understanding that there was apparently no law enforcement professional who—using an accepted protocol, would step into a case like this and based on experience, intuition, and determination—could stop a Swango in his tracks.

Even if the brass at OSU was inclined to discover the truth, there was no expertise available to them either in-house or in local law enforcement. I was exploring unknown territory by trying to build a case. That understanding encouraged me to keep going. There had to be some way to stop the madman.

This would not be a case of paper trails. Even while my team gathered more and more anecdotal evidence, I understood it would never be enough. I was going to have to solve the puzzle of physical evidence. "There must be a way," I would say to anyone who would listen.

I was constantly talking about the Swango case with my family and friends. We could be talking about sports, school, or business, and his name would come up. Believe me, they were never bored. Everyone was as astounded as I was that this monster was never caught and was still on the loose, probably preying on the weak.

I would talk to doctors and search the library for books on poison and chemicals that could cause death. My staff kidded me about my growing obsession with the case. Even before Swango, they said I looked more like a doctor than a detective; now they started calling me *Doctor Bruce*, a nickname that has stuck with me ever since. I am proud of it.

I figured he must know which drugs could be administered and which could kill but not be traced or determined at an autopsy. I accepted that if I ever were to make a case against Swango, I would need the help of experts, medical examiners, chemists, and psychiatrists. Tom and I were expert detectives, but a jury would not accept our testimony about the properties of arsenic in ant poison.

I did not realize it at the time, but subconsciously, I was creating a protocol to catch medical serial killers. As one year became two and we still did not have our hands on Swango, Tom and I became more and more obsessed with the case. We talked about it over coffee, lunch, and after every briefing on our other cases. But as long as the FBI froze us out, all we could do was continue to prepare for the day Swango was in handcuffs.

The dossier continued to grow. We learned "Double O Swango" was released on good behavior in 1987 after serving two and a half years. To make ends meet, he crisscrossed the country taking low-paying jobs as a medical technician. He found work as a counselor at the Career Development Center in Newport News, Virginia. There he made colleagues' skin crawl when they found him working on a scrapbook about disasters with many deaths. I wondered if the scrapbook was in his room at Stony Brook. The room I was not allowed to search.

Valery picked up the trail of records again, discovering that in 1991, Swango was taking a refresher course at Riverside Hospital in Newport News, Virginia. While there, he met a beautiful twenty-six-year-old nurse named Kristin Kinney who was known for her professional nursing, trusting personality, and gorgeous red hair. The two became an item.

About a year later, Swango contacted the University of South Dakota Sanford School of Medicine about joining its medical residency program. This time, he employed another of his skills to convince them his criminal past should not preclude his hiring. He forged two important documents. The first was a fact sheet from the Illinois Department of Corrections, which falsely stated he had been convicted of a misdemeanor for being in a barroom brawl and received six months in prison. Next, he forged a "Restoration of Rights" letter from Virginia Governor Gerald Baliles, falsely claiming he had restored all of Swango's civil rights. The letter stated that his friends and colleagues had vouched for him having had led an "exemplary lifestyle" after serving his time on the misdemeanor conviction. These were the same documents he would subsequently show to the Stony Brook administration.

He then went through a battery of interviews regarding his qualifications but, incredibly, no one questioned his story about the conviction or wondered why he had a letter from the governor of Virginia when his conviction was in Illinois.

Throughout the interview process, we discovered that no one apparently thought it necessary to contact OSU or law enforcement back in Quincy, Illinois to confirm Swango's dismissal of his crime as a mere barroom brawl. I found that incredible. Had I been so lax in my career about checking out the backgrounds of job applicants for the Air Force or the VA, I would have found myself running a freight elevator at a lonely VA outpost in Alaska. But Swango got the job and began working at Sanford University of South Dakota Medical Center in Sioux Falls.

Swango celebrated by asking Kinney to marry him. She happily accepted and agreed to follow him to Sioux Falls.

Tom and I found Kinney's mother, Sharon Cooper, and with her help, were able to form an impression of the relationship between Swango and the young nurse whose friends called her "K.K." Of all the people touched by Swango, none of them had such a profound effect on me as Kinney. She was perfect prey for a predator.

She was searching for a relationship following a divorce and was vulnerable to the charming, persuasive killer. She did not know it, but to Swango, she was just another victim.

At first all was fine. Kinney's parents adored and admired the young, handsome doctor. Although they were troubled by the gaps in his background, they initially accepted Swango as a great mate for their beloved daughter. Perhaps now, they felt she could find the happiness she deserved.

Incredibly, despite his questionable background, Swango was selected for the South Dakota residency program and was assigned to the outpatient clinic of the Sioux Falls VA Medical Center in June 1992. Kinney followed him to Sioux Falls, where she was hired as a registered nurse at the Royal C. Johnson Veterans Memorial Medical Center.

Residents from the university rotate through the VA, as the Stony Brook residents rotated through Northport, and before long Swango and Kinney were both working at Royal C. Johnson Memorial Medical Center.

Members of the staff there told us that Swango was one of the best emergency room doctors they ever had. They said if a patient coded, it was Swango whom they hoped would respond. Everything seemed to be falling in place for nurse Kinney and her doctor fiancé.

Swango became so confident that his past was buried behind him that he applied for membership in the American Medical Association (AMA). This was a rare blunder for the con artist. The AMA, unlike seemingly everyone else with whom Swango dealt over the years, did not routinely accept anyone just because they had a convincing story. They did a thorough background check and uncovered Swango's criminal past. This time he could not explain his way out of it.

At that time, *20/20* repeated its story about Swango, the one that contained the jailhouse interview with John Stossel. It was seen by most of the staff at Sanford, including Kristen Kinney. Now, everyone was suspicious of Swango. At parties, they watched him closely if he moved near the punch bowl. Sanford, looking to avoid any scandal, fired Swango.

Sadly, Kinney became the butt of jokes around the hospital and the small town. One radio station famously concocted a cruel song to the tune of "Rudolph the Red-Nosed Reindeer," and played it without mercy.

"Swango the troubled doctor
USD say out he goes
And if you saw his rap sheet
All of us would say 'Oh no!'"

It was more cruel than clever, and Kinney certainly did not deserve the humiliation it brought to her.

Rather than continue the humiliation and her nursing work at Royal C. Johnson without her fiancé, Kinney moved back to her parents in Virginia. She told friends in Sanford she was suffering from devastating headaches and feared Swango might be poisoning her.

Back home, and away from Swango, the headaches eased. But Swango continued to pursue her. He called and wrote and professed his undying love for her, swearing he would never harm her.

Poor Kristen, they were separated by a thousand miles, but she could not shake her fear of the monster. After about four months of their separation, she walked to a nearby park and shot herself in the chest. The cause of death was suicide by gunshot. There was no mention of Swango in the coroner's report.

The unfortunate young woman left a note behind in her apartment, addressed to her mother, father, and her fiancé that read as follows:

> "*I love you both so much. I just don't want to be here anymore. Just found day-to-day living a constant struggle with my thoughts. I'd say I'm sorry but I'm not. I feel a sense of peace, "peace of mind" I've been looking for, It's nice.*"

An addendum addressed to Swango read, "*I love you more! You're the most precious man I've ever known.*"

Her parents viewed Swango as a torturer and blamed him for their daughter's suicide. They believed he was trying to kill her. They would get no argument from me.

Kinney's body was cremated. However, I was told by a VA contact in Sanford that just before the cremation, her mother saved a lock of her striking red hair and put it in an envelope.

I told Valery to locate that lock of hair.

It sounds unbelievable but at this time in 1993, Swango convinced psychiatrists at the Health Science School for Medicine at Stony Brook University, that the nature of his arrest and conviction in Illinois had been so menial as to not constitute any reason to deny his entry into their program. He was accepted.

But the television program Doctor Thomesen saw continued to be Swango's nemesis. Sharon Cooper also saw the program and then did some detective work of her own to learn Swango's whereabouts. She convinced the dean at Sanford to contact officials at Stony Brook. It was only hours after I questioned Swango when the Stony Brook dean and the head of the psychiatry unit questioned Swango, and fired him. The same year, the dean and the head of psychiatry were fired by Stony Brook.

But there were still no crimes at Northport linked to him. No suspicious deaths, no poisoning of paramedics, no girlfriends shooting themselves in the chest, and leaving a suicide note.

Then, finally, Swango was located. I would get my chance to nail him.

CHAPTER 6

Nailed in Chicago

"The dead cannot cry out for justice.
It is a duty of the living to do so for them."

—LOIS McMASTER BUJOLD

Time passed and Swango became a household name in my office. As head of the investigation, it was my duty to keep the team's eye on the prize. I called on several agents, including Tom and Samantha, to make follow-up phone calls and keep tabs on media in Ohio and Illinois and, of course, the cable documentary channels.

We had a mini-disaster when a water pipe in the ceiling burst and flooded the section of the office where we stored Swango's paperwork. Much of it was spared because it was on high shelves, but much was soaked in wet piles on the floor and knee-deep water. Tom went downstairs to his car and retrieved his firefighter gear. I rolled up my pants to my knee and waded into the mess in a desperate attempt to save as much of the crucial paperwork as I could. Then Tom showed up wearing his firefighter's boots and pants and sloshed through the muck to save the day. He recovered almost all the significant work.

A few days after that, on July 23, 1997, Tom received a call from Assistant United States Attorney Cecilia Gardner. She was asking for his assistance on the case.

Tom was bursting with energy when he walked through my door to deliver the news.

"Boss, they got him. Immigration nabbed him at Chicago O'Hare."

At first I didn't make the connection. "Who'd they get? Immigration?"

"It's Swango. I got a call from an AUSA. She's asking for your help. Customs stopped Swango coming in from Africa at O'Hare on an outstanding FBI warrant for fraud. They're holding him and need our help in filling in the details.

"This attorney, Cecilia Gardner, says the original agent on the case has been transferred and they need us to fill in the blanks."

Tom was breathless and I was speechless. I mumbled my surprise.

"Fraud?" I asked. I thought the Bureau had rejected our view that we pursue fraud charges. Well, what do you know! They took my advice but did not have the courtesy to even let me in on it. No surprise there. Anyway, we're back in the game and we're locked and loaded.

"If he was in Africa," I asked Tom, "how did they get him at O'Hare?"

"All they told me was that he was in Zimbabwe and was leaving to take a doctor's position in Saudi Arabia. Apparently, he had to touch base in the US to pick up a Saudi Arabian visa before going there and the feds had previously flagged his passport. They must have known he was in Africa."

Well that was news to me. What else did they know that they did not share? Now they were asking us to share the VA files. If this was a way to nail the bastard I had been thinking about for more than two years, then I would not let the pettiness of the FBI stand in the way. I told Tom to gather our team for a strategy meeting in about an hour while I called the suits in DC.

As soon as Tom left my office, I took a deep breath and took out a fresh legal pad from my drawer. I wrote out a few notes that covered our Swango-related activities over the years and bases I knew we had to revisit. I listed the Quincy paramedics, OSU investigation, Kristin Kinney's hair, Sanford nurses, and a lot more people with whom we needed to reconnect. Then I called David Gamble in Washington. He was the man I had replaced as special agent in charge in New York when he was promoted to a position in DC His boss was Michael Costello, a former DEA agent who had a degree in pharmacy. Being a former DEA guy, Costello was very aggressive about investigations. Gamble was more conservative.

Together, they were an efficient team and over the past three years, never questioned the resources I was putting into the Swango case. They had been embarrassed by the screwup at Stony Brook and, though it was not the VA's fault, they felt Swango's ability to practice medicine at the Northport VA facility was inexcusable.

There were some rumblings at the highest levels of the VA that we were working outside the mandate of the inspector general's office in pursuing a murder investigation, but the general counsel wrote a memo supporting us.

Gamble gave me the go-ahead to do whatever I needed to help with the fraud case, then continue to determine if Swango had actually killed veterans in Northport.

A few minutes later Costello, having been briefed by Gamble, called to offer his support. With his degree in pharmacy, he understood how chemicals can be used to kill. He then gave me the most significant advice I was ever to receive in my career.

He suggested I get in touch with Doctor Michael Baden, the former chief medical examiner (ME) for New York City and renowned forensic pathologist. He was the host of the HBO documentary series, *Autopsy*.

"Trust me, you'll love the guy and if Swango killed at Northport, he will know how to prove it," Costello said.

I had heard of Baden but honestly had not thought about seeking his help before Costello suggested it. Of course, it made sense and I asked my secretary to try to locate the famous doctor.

When my small group gathered in my office, I explained my strategy of putting Swango away for a few years on the fraud charges to give us the needed time to pursue murder charges. It was the same advice I offered Loretta Lynch three years earlier when I was sent packing by the FBI.

I told Tom to get back to AUSA Cecilia Gardner's office and arrange a meeting, but first I told him I wanted to meet Baden. Hopefully the legendary ME would hear me out.

I tracked Baden down through the current NYC Medical Examiner's Office. He took my phone call and was encouraging from the moment I introduced myself. I quickly told him what I was trying to do: prove a doctor had murdered some patients in a VA medical center. He said I should come up to Albany, New York, where he was serving as codirector of the New York State Police Medicolegal Investigation Unit. I had never heard of the unit, but the title indicated it was just what I was looking for. He told me he was working with

Doctor Lowell Levine, a forensic dentist. The two traveled all over the world performing autopsies and conducting forensic examinations.

He said he would see me as soon as I could get there, so we set a date for three days later. That evening I got a copy of a book Baden coauthored—*Unnatural Death: Confessions of a Medical Examiner,* which I managed to read before the meeting. It was fascinating.

So when Tom and I walked in to Baden's office in Albany, I was surprised to find him as a larger-than-life character. I was expecting a professor type, small and disheveled, but he was about six feet two inches, in good shape, and well-dressed. He had huge hands that I noticed were hairless. I had this thought that the hair might have been destroyed by chemicals he used in his work. He exuded a star-like quality and aura that made you feel like you were in the presence of someone special.

After introductions, we quickly got down to business. Baden asked me direct questions about what we knew, what we suspected, and what we could prove.

I filled him in on the fraud aspects, the meeting at Northport, and the suspicious history we had dug up, including the suicide of Kristin Kinney. Tom relayed his interviews with the paramedics whom Swango poisoned and the subsequent prison conviction.

It was clear, we told him, that Swango was suspected of killing patients at OSU, and we were prepared to rip into records at Northport to find suspicious deaths.

But, I had to admit when he asked if we could prove anything such as murder, my answer was "No!" But my answer did not faze him. He was expecting it. He understood I had little experience in homicide, and just said, "Well, that's what I'm here for."

He said he was intrigued with the idea of helping us, wanted to review whatever medical records we had immediately available, and would like to meet with Gardner as soon as possible. He was aboard!

That made my day. I was thrilled to have an internationally-renowned forensic pathologist as a mentor, as I further evolved into a homicide detective!

I hit a bump in the road when I called the New York State Police bosses and formally requested Baden's help. After all, he was on their payroll. Surprisingly, they refused my request, saying they did not want to get involved with the FBI, who they expected would be taking the lead on the investigation.

When I relayed this to Baden, he told me he could not resist such a challenging case and did not care whom he pissed off in order to get the job done. He said he would help us on his own without state police involvement.

A few days later, Baden joined Tom and I in Gardner's office. The doctor agreed with our strategy. He wanted to select certain cases from the files that seemed most suspicious and then exhume those bodies for forensic autopsies.

I exchanged glances with Tom while Baden spoke. We knew we could never have made a case for doing what he proposed. It was so far out of our expertise that we would have been laughed out of the office.

But Gardner was not as impressed as we were. She listened quietly and then asked Baden to leave the room while the rest of us discussed his proposal.

Always the gentleman, Baden rose from his chair opposite Gardner's desk and said, "I'm old enough to accept rejection," as he walked into the waiting room outside the door.

As soon as the door closed, Gardner tore into the famous doctor. She berated his reputation as a media hound who could not be trusted as a team player. She said she would not work with him and that we should find someone else.

Well, there was no chance of that happening. I was sold on Baden and prepared to bring him aboard without her blessing. In fact, I had already shared the medical records of the deceased patient with him. Our visit to Gardner was a courtesy to keep her in the loop. Now I was sorry I did it. If she gave me a hard time as we moved along, I would take it up with DC.

When Tom and I walked into the waiting room, I shook Baden's hand and said, "Welcome aboard, let's get to work."

Gardner would prove to be no trouble.

Events now began moving quickly. Through Baden, I was introduced to a world of forensic experts including Doctor Fredric Rieders, founder of National Medical Services, one of the most advanced forensic and clinical toxicology labs in the world; Doctor Henry Lee, the world-renowned forensic scientist, who testified in the OJ Simpson trial; and Special Agent Brian Donnelly of the FBI. Donnelly had a PhD in toxicology and was earlier assigned to the FBI laboratory in Washington, DC As a result of a managerial shake-up of the lab, he was reassigned to the FBI office in New Haven, Connecticut.

But first on the agenda was preparing a four-count indictment charging Swango with fraud in lying to Stony Brook University, which enabled his assignment to a VA medical center. That was in the jurisdiction of the US Attorney for the Eastern District of New York. In addition, the four-count indictment charged Swango with illegally dispensing controlled substances. He was not properly licensed although he lied on his application to the contrary. We had that much solid. I was certain we would at least be able to hold Swango in prison for a couple of years while we prepared the homicide case.

In March 1998, while he was stewing in the federal lockup in Chicago, Swango was informed of the hard evidence against him for the fraud committed on Long Island, and that an investigation was underway into his activities in Zimbabwe.

Five months later, he pled guilty to defrauding the government and was sentenced to three and a half years in prison. The sentencing judge, as the judge in Quincy, Illinois, had done, ordered that Swango not be allowed to work in the prison kitchen or deliver food to inmates, and not have any involvement in preparing or delivering drugs.

I don't believe Swango was concerned about our now very active investigation at Northport, but he was troubled by the thought we would uncover devilish doings in Africa, which convinced him to take the plea. He was hoping that while behind bars, we would lose interest in pursuing anything else and the case would all go away.

He could not have been more wrong.

CHAPTER 7

Angels and Autopsies

"Never ask a barber if you need a haircut; you
never ask a forensic pathologist if an exhumation is
needed."

—DOCTOR MICHAEL BADEN

With Swango cooling his heels in jail, it fell on me to
put my money where my mouth was. We had a team
in place, led by Doctor Baden, which consisted of a group of
handpicked nurses who became known as "Bruce's Angels,"
FBI agents, technicians, and scientists.

Most important to our overall success was the assignment
of three forensic nurses: Shirley Henley, Patricia Christ, and
Linda Delong, all of whom I requested from the Office of
Healthcare Inspections based in DC. They had diverse training
and education, and they proved to be professionals who were
indispensable to our overall effort. Once a week for almost a
year, they traveled to the Jacob K. Javits Federal Building, near
the Federal Courthouse in Manhattan, to conduct a review of
147 patients who received treatment from Swango. Their main

task was to review each medical record to assure timeliness and safety of appropriate patient care.

The three women worked out of a windowless twenty by fifteen foot "war room" surrounded by medical records and documents lining the walls. Each of these items was a potential piece of damaging evidence against Swango.

Medical records and documents were collected from the Department of Veterans Affairs in Northport, NY; Ohio State University Hospital; and Zimbabwe, Africa. They revealed a pattern of behavior by Doctor Swango at his patients' bedsides: he entered their rooms by himself, drew the curtains, and administered lethal injections of a paralyzing medication.

The rest of the team worked out of a small conference room that the Suffolk County Medical Examiner in New York was kind enough to lend us for the duration of the investigation. I don't think he realized how many people would be involved and how long it would take us. We were all paid our regular salaries from our parent agencies; Rieders, a civilian, was paid by my office. It was crowded and intense, but I was very excited and eager to get to work each day. On those days when I thought we might be just spinning our wheels, I would get a boost of energy watching the team focus on the tasks at hand. There was no goofing off. It was a dedicated team.

We also had some new technology going for us. At one point, as we began in earnest to review records, more than one thousand items were piled on my usually neat-as-a pin-desk. It was a daunting task staring me in the face every morning when I reported to the office. Thankfully, a clerical assistant suggested we employ a new computer program recently made available by the VA. I had no experience with the program, which was known as Analyst's Notebook, but was eager to give it a try. I would appreciate any help I could get with that pile of paper.

Without the help of that program, we may never have been able to stop Swango.

My clerical staff and I entered large amounts of data, such as patients' names, conditions, and doctor's visits. The software sorted it all and produced several charts and graphs, which were used as evidence to convict Swango.

For instance, we learned from Analyst's Notebook the names of patients Swango was seeing at particular times. It helped us focus on who his victims were, and which patients dodged his bullets never even knowing they were in danger.

The VA, as well as many other law enforcement agencies throughout the country, eventually made Analyst's Notebook a standard part of their arsenal. It was great knowing we had identified a new tool we could use to catch monsters like Swango.

For months, Baden had been conducting a master's class on forensic pathology. He taught us the procedures of how to find traces of drugs in the bodies of the victims we intended to exhume. They all died on Swango's watch. He had opportunity behind the murder curtain with victims and he had access to certain drugs. By this time, we knew his motive was the joy of killing. The identity of the victim really did not matter to him.

The legendary medical examiner expected to find traces of epinephrine, which temporarily speeds up the heart and can kill if the dose is too high, and succinylcholine, which causes paralysis. Around the office we called it "sucs."

I was especially bothered by the use of epinephrine as a murder weapon. My son struggled with serious asthma attacks as a teenager and we made many emergency trips to the

ER for an injection of this drug. Epinephrine was a miracle drug for us and saved his life on at least one occasion. It depressed me to think of the use Swango found for it. Baden theorized he would first inject the epinephrine, wait a few minutes, and then add the sucs to the mix. It would not be an instant death.

Our conversations would often turn to motive. We were all familiar with the "Angel of Death" scenario. That is when doctors, nurses, or other medical professionals find a way to relieve their patients from horrible suffering by killing them. They view it as an act of humanity and some will argue the concept should be legal, like assisted suicide, in certain places.

But as we peeled away the layers of information we had on Swango, the "Angel of Death" argument ran out of steam.

"This guy just killed for the fun of it," Valery would say. I agreed with him. And while nurses who worked with him in Ohio told investigators they believed he stole money and jewelry from the purses of his victims, we never believed money was his motive. Everyone on our team eventually came to believe Swango was a madman, killing for the joy of killing.

We examined the many dozens of victim files of that fit our strategy for catching a killer. We first looked at veterans who died unexpectedly. They might have been in the hospital for relatively minor surgery, or with an ailment that had been treated, and they were on the way to recovery. We looked for "heart attack" as a cause of death because essentially it was common and probably not questioned. One thing we checked was the time of death. It is unusual for patients to die during the evening. Most died in late afternoon. I don't know why, but that is a fact. Of course, a crucial criterion was if Swango was the last doctor to pay a visit to their hospital bed. Was Swango the last to pull the curtain around them before the patient died? The hospital records could reveal that information.

Baden explained to our group that when we narrowed the field, we would select the most likely cases for exhumation. The thought gave me the creeps. Of course, absent a confession or hidden camera video, there could be no other way to determine the cause of death. I also imagined that it would take a court order and the cooperation of families to take these men from their "final resting places."

I naïvely asked Baden if he thought it was absolutely necessary to exhume these men. The answer was Baden's slogan: "Never ask a barber if you need a haircut; you never ask a forensic pathologist if you need an exhumation."

Of course, we would need to get to those bodies. After weeks of pouring over records, we decided on the five people whose bodies fit our criteria. They were:

- Dominic Buffalino, a longtime Suffolk County official who was on the road to recovery from a bout with pneumonia. He died unexpectedly during Swango's first day on the job at Northport;
- George Siano, who was winning his battle with cancer when he died suddenly;
- Barron Harris, who became paralyzed after Swango treated him. He complained to staff that someone was trying to kill him, but no one believed him. He subsequently died;
- Aldo Serini, sixty-two, who was being treated for respiratory problems; and
- Thomas Sammarco, seventy-three, who was being tested for open heart surgery, only to be murdered.

The next few weeks, we were occupied with getting court orders, so the cemetery would allow us to dig up the graves, and of course we needed to get the permission of the families involved.

The day before the exhumation, I learned that a nurse at Northport saw Swango sitting for more than an hour on a radiator in the curtained-off area of a woman who had recovered from surgery and was ready to leave the intensive care unit (ICU). The next doctor to check on the woman found her dead. That was just how I envisioned Swango at work.

It was a sunny, spring day when we went out to the VA cemetery in Farmingdale, New York. A small group of my team and some family members of the deceased gathered on a cemetery road to await Baden. Not a shovelful of dirt would be turned without his presence. It was a tense, quiet scene. We did not want anything to go wrong that might endanger the investigation, and at the same time, we were afraid of disrespecting the victim and his family.

An exhumation is like no other event I know. It is the process of disturbing the dead. The phrase "rest in peace" no longer applies because after months or even several years after a body is placed in the ground, law enforcement may discover a need to disrupt a body everyone had assumed would remain untouched forever.

The condition of the coffin depends on several factors, especially the materials used for its construction and whether it is encased in a liner. The water table is an important consideration as well, since sometimes coffins that are removed are full of water and the body nearly floats away. Some remains look remarkably well preserved, even after long periods of time, while others, even after a few months in the ground, look unrecognizable. Dental records and personal items known to have been buried with the deceased are used for identification. Even though we had a map of where the person was buried, and of course, there was a grave marker, the body could have shifted underground, or some other mistake at the time of burial could have occurred and we could be examining the wrong body. Soil samples were taken to determine if any chemicals found in the body were present in the soil.

One of the county sheriff deputies who I had gotten to know stood beside me on the road. In a very low voice, he relayed an incident that he was involved in when he worked in Brooklyn. He was doing security at an exhumation the Brooklyn District Attorney (DA) had organized, much the same as his job was this day, just different jurisdictions.

He said the Brooklyn event was a big story and there were reporters gathered around the gravesite and news helicopters overhead.

He told me that as the casket was raised from the grave, it began to break apart. It was rotted with age, and weeds and roots protruded from it. It was right out of a horror movie. Then the remains slid out one end and dangled half-in, half-out, while the workmen lifted it on to solid ground.

The deputy had my attention as he described how everyone stood in horror, the helicopter's engine drowning out gagged responses.

"They got the job done," he said. "And the television station did not show it."

Suddenly, Baden pulled up in his old Mercedes, which made me think of the television detective Columbo arriving at a crime scene in his beat-up old junker. Baden told the ground crew they could begin.

There were no helicopters circling overhead but I still prayed nothing would fall apart as the crew shoveled away the moist black dirt packed around the wooden coffin. It was a relatively recent grave and when the casket was raised by pulley from the ground, I was relieved to see that it was not damaged. It was easily transferred to the back of a county vehicle to be driven to the medical examiner's laboratory. The morgue.

As soon as the grave was empty, Doctor Baden, who always wore a suit and tie, did something that gained him the admiration of the entire team. No sooner was the casket loaded into the back of the morgue van than Baden jumped into the grave. He got down on a knee, took an envelope out of his suit jacket pocket, and collected soil samples. He carefully marked each envelope. For him, it was just another day at the office. When he appeared to be finished, I walked to the edge of the grave and reached my hand down to help him back to the surface.

I asked what that was all about. "We'll need to analyze this dirt. If there is a trace of any chemical that might have killed our victim, it will be very significant evidence," he explained. I had a fitting thought right then that this was the guy I would trust with anything. I always admired people who were experts at their work. He was curious and tireless, and most of all, he inspired the confidence in all of us that we were doing something important.

In all, before we were done, we exhumed five bodies without incident. However, we found one naked in his coffin. The jewelry he was buried with, including a medal he was awarded in combat, was missing. That was embarrassing and inexcusable. I told Tom to assign an agent to investigate what happened to his clothes and jewelry.

When we got back to the lab, an FBI profiler who had been assigned to the case was waiting to brief me. I hadn't met him before and it was the first I knew of his assignment. I offered him some iced tea (an inside joke for Tom's sake) and the three of us sat at a table in a small coffee room. He told us that Swango was probably a serial killer and probably killed the people we identified. He found some research on what he called "Medical Serial Killers (MSKs), and assumed, as we had assumed, that many got away with murder over the years because there was little inclination on the part of hospitals and medical schools to expose them. There was also no proven scientific method to convict them.

The MSKs are psychopathic killers. They kill for the pleasure of watching someone die and they kill for monetary gain. One doctor in England, for instance, added himself added to his patient's life insurance policies. He would then kill them and collect the insurance. One killed because she got off on calling the victim's family to break the news that their loved one had passed away.

An FBI agent told a newspaper in Illinois that Swango displayed characteristics associated with "organizational murderers," such as "above average intelligence, sexual and social competence, and a controlled mood during the crime."

But we still had no hard evidence either in Ohio or Illinois that Swango killed any of his patients.

It was always my premise that if he was willing to poison people, he was willing to kill them, even accidentally from too much poison. It was just luck that the paramedic back in Quincy survived his donuts. So "probably" was not enough. Although this profiler would make a compelling expert witness, I was going to need more. I could not take a "probably" to court. We needed to be certain. However, we did like the label "MSKs," and from that meeting on, it stuck as our abbreviation for Swango. We would prove he was an MSK.

The same day I also met Bob Golden, an investigator at the Suffolk County ME's office, who said he notified the FBI four years earlier about his suspicions that patients at Northport were being murdered. He said they ignored him.

A few hours after we dug up the first body, Baden invited me to watch him perform the autopsy. As curious as I was to see the doctor in action, I was filled with apprehension about being so close to a body being cut up. And I did not know what useful purpose my being there would serve. But how could I say no? I was the boss and needed to lead. And Baden clearly loved to show off his expertise knowing he would shock some people and even make some gag, but eventually everyone came to respect him for his desire to share his knowledge.

One of "Bruce's Angels" fitted me with a doctor's smock and handed me a small bottle of Vicks VapoRub. She said I should rub some over my upper lip, under my nose. "It will help with the smell," she said. Then she led me down a corridor to the autopsy room where Baden was waiting to begin his work.

As we entered the room, the first thing I reacted to was the smell. Despite the Vicks ointment, I was immediately sickened by the unique smell. It was the smell of death: disinfectant, chemicals, and body odor. Not the body odor we are accustomed to in a locker room, but odor caused by the gore that results from cutting open a body, removing organs, and using a saw to get to the innards of an arm, leg, or some other part that is protected by bone. The staff calls it the "odor of decay." You would have to swim in an ocean of *Vicks* to escape it.

An NYPD detective, who lived near us in Plainview, once told me a story about a New York City medical examiner.

"When the ME was pissed at the brass upstairs for some reason or other, he would open the vents in the autopsy room and let the death odor seep throughout the building. It was disgusting."

I hadn't thought about that since, but now I knew what the detective was talking about. Everything about the room turned my stomach. It was like a chamber of torture and horrors, especially the instruments. In the middle of the room, under bright light, the naked body of the deceased was waiting for Baden to do his work. On a table alongside, there were a variety of saws; some were called Stryker saws for ripping bone, and others were used for cutting through cartilage, muscle, and tissue. There were scalpels, knives, suturing materials, instruments for spreading ribs or organs, and various vessels and containers used to capture body fluids and hold organs.

There was a sink at the end of the table connected to a holding tank to collect the fluids that would have to be saved for later study. In those fluids and body parts, Baden believed we would find our evidence of poison. A microphone hung over the stainless-steel slab, so the medical examiner could provide a running commentary on what he was doing. I was fascinated and revolted by the process all at the same time.

When Baden made his first cut, a Y-shaped incision down the center of the body, I had to control myself from tossing my lunch. Once I fought that impulse, I got under control and was able to concentrate. That's when I first realized how cold it was in the room. It was just a little above freezing.

I watched as Baden removed the heart from the body and walked around the table to stand directly in front of me. He patiently showed me the heart, turning it slowly in his hands to show me why he believed this particular victim did not die from natural causes. He said the heart did not appear to show damage from disease or injury. He said the arteries, veins, and valves all looked pretty strong to him.

He described the difference between natural death and homicide. He told me "a natural death is an event akin to shutting off a fan where the blades gradually stop spinning. But our victims died much the way a light bulb is turned off. One moment it is bright and one moment later it is dark."

Those moments of education marked the few days spent working over the bodies. Everyone who encountered Baden learned something. All the knowledge was aimed at putting Swango in a place where he would not be able to harm another person.

After a week of autopsies, Baden determined that none of the individuals we selected had died from natural causes. He believed they must have been poisoned and examination of the tissues he removed would prove that. This was not as easy as Baden made it sound.

In all our interviews with detectives, prosecutors, and nurses, especially at OSU, when prosecution was given serious consideration, we were told the bottom line was that it was almost impossible to find traces of certain drugs used as a weapon of death. And these drugs, because they had vital legitimate uses, were readily available on crash carts and in hospital drug lockers.

You could prove Swango had access to drugs that could do the job. You could prove he had opportunity either when alone with a patient or when he was involved in an emergency situation. But unless you could follow the trail of the drugs, from the hospital pharmacy to Swango's hands, and finally into the victim, you were dead in the water as far as a conviction was concerned.

But we had a couple of weapons our colleagues around the country did not have. We had Baden and a remarkable man he brought on the team, named Doctor Fredric Rieders.

Doctor Rieders was an internationally renowned forensic toxicologist. He utilized a machine called the High Performance Liquid Chromatography Tandem Mass Spectrometry. About as big as a 1950s television console, it could test tissue to see if there were traces of drugs that should not be in the system according to the patient's medical records.

Rieders served in the Army during World War II and had a loyalty to his fellow veterans that I found admirable. It gave him a special appreciation of the case. The process he developed to search for certain substances in embalmed tissue was time-consuming and very expensive. It was on the cutting edge of forensic pathology and therefore controversial in the field. Many scientists insisted it could not be done. I got some advice suggesting I not employ him for this case. But Baden had faith in him and I was not afraid to push the envelope. This whole investigation was about envelope-pushing as far as my office was concerned. We were not exactly the NYPD homicide squad.

Baden took the tissue he thought would be the best to Doctor Rieders, who put his machine to work. It took several weeks of careful examination, but eventually he was willing to testify that there were traces of succinylcholine and epinephrine in three of the five patients whose bodies we recovered. Doctor Rieders' lab work showed these patients had one or both of these drugs in them, and Baden agreed that their deaths were consistent with that poisoning. That made whoever put those drugs into their bodies a murderer. That was Swango.

Now we were ready to bring our evidence to James Conway and Gary Brown, the Assistant US Attorneys assigned as the prosecutors, and get a grand jury to begin hearing our evidence. A murder indictment was in the cards.

CHAPTER 8

Africa

"Whenever a doctor cannot do good,
he must be kept from doing harm."

—HIPPOCRATES

It took us almost three years to get to the point of presenting evidence to the grand jury about the Northport murders. During that time, the FBI was busy investigating what exactly Swango was doing in Africa, after he fled from Northport.

Unbeknownst to me, AUSA Cecilia Gardner learned Swango, using forged documents, obtained a position at Mnene Hospital in Zimbabwe. She led a team to Africa and met with officials there about Swango's status. Apparently, she accomplished little on her secret trip because one year later, in November 1995, Swango was arrested and charged with poisoning patients he treated at that hospital. But before he could be tried, he escaped to Zambia, where he hid out for a year.

In March 1997, Swango applied for a job in Dhahran, Saudi Arabia, using those forged documents and a contrived résumé. But he could not travel to Saudi Arabia without first touching down in the US and having his passport stamped. When he did, that customs and immigration officers were waiting to handcuff him and lead him away to the federal lockup in Chicago.

While we were digging up bodies and examining the remains, the US Attorney organized another trip to Africa. Although it was a joint investigation, he wanted to dictate who from my office would go with them. The agent organizing the trip had the gall to tell Samantha Lockery that if she were to go to Africa, she would be left at the airport on her own and would only delay the FBI in its work. Hearing this, Tom refused to go at all. I agreed with Tom. To me this was intolerable. I can only attribute it to some ignorant male chauvinism. Tom was right to insist on Samantha being treated like the competent dedicated agent she had proven herself to be.

I was the guy on our team who knew how to handle the brass. I went directly to one of the most senior agents in charge of the FBI's New York office and explained the untenable situation. I told him no one knew the Swango case as well as we did and to be shut out at this time was unprofessional and beyond reason. I was prepared to take my argument to DC if necessary.

Well, I did not have to go further. My argument fell on reasonable ears and the word was passed down to include Samantha, Brian Donnelly, and a calmed-down Tom on the traveling team. I was certain Brian and Tom would make sure Samantha was treated with the professional courtesy she deserved. We discovered that Swango, on the run, proved to be as cunning and amoral as ever. After he fled Northport and hid in Georgia, he contacted an agency that found English-speaking doctors for work in developing countries. Using his usual file of forged documents and résumés, he landed a spot in the remote Mnene Lutheran Christian Hospital staffed by Lutheran nurses in Mnene, Zimbabwe.

The people in Mnene who hired Swango and then assigned him to cases were more than eager to speak with our team. They said they were suspicious that such a sophisticated doctor who worked in top-rated American hospitals would want to practice in their ill-equipped facility in the middle of nowhere. But the smooth-talking con artist impressed them. He convinced them his heart was devoted to helping the less fortunate. They remained skeptical but American doctors were hard to come by, and they brought him aboard despite their misgivings.

The director of the mission station in Mnene was Doctor Christopher Zshiri, a man who was truly devoted to helping the less fortunate. Early on during Swango's orientation period, Doctor Zshiri noticed the American lacked certain skills and was not interested in treating minor ailments that were so commonplace in his hospital. Burns, splinters, cysts, and infections did not interest him. Zshiri believed that Swango, who pretended to be a neurosurgeon, was just unfamiliar with this basic care. He decided to transfer him to Mpilo Hospital, a more advanced facility in Bulawayo, Zimbabwe, as part of an internship.

After five months at Mpilo, Swango had become friendly with the locals and doctors, and had impressed many with his energy and verve. He was then able to return to Mnene.

Doctor Zshiri told our team that soon after his arrival, patients began to die unexpectedly for suspicious reasons. "People with simple illnesses or who were on the road to recovery kept dying on his ward," said a nurse who was apprehensive about talking to our investigators because she feared reprisals from her bosses.

It was learned that Swango kept a private supply of drugs in a refrigerator in his home and carried two syringes on his rounds. He would hide one syringe in his pocket and hold another in his hand. One night, it was alleged, he used this hidden medication on an unsuspecting patient named Kennias Muzeziwa, fifty-six, a peasant farmer, who was recuperating after having most of his left foot amputated due to infection. The wound was virtually healed, and he was awaiting a prosthesis promised by a Swedish charity.

When my team visited him in his mud hut, he recounted that one night in the hospital, he was awakened by someone pulling down his pajama bottom. When he looked up from his pillow he saw "Doctor Mike with an injection, which he put in my buttocks. He then waved goodbye and walked away."

Muzeziwa felt faint and tried to call for help but remembered he could not breath. Finally, a nurse heard his weak cry and rushed to his side. He whispered to her what had happened. The nurse found the top from a syringe under his bed.

Swango was confronted but arrogantly denied the entire episode, claiming a similar charge was brought against him at another African hospital. The nurses complained to my team that they could do nothing.

Muzeziwa lived through his ordeal but had to have his leg amputated up to the knee, which made it impossible for him to continue as a farmer and doomed him and his wife to a life of abject poverty.

Swango was suspended but no proof that he had done anything wrong could be determined because of inadequate investigations. Swango hired a lawyer to help him get more clinical work. However, a respected surgeon reported to authorities that he often found Swango snooping around the wards and ICU even when he was off-duty. Again, the surgeon had great suspicions about the untimely deaths but no physical evidence that could connect Swango.

While in Mnene, a woman named Edith Ngwenya, who washed and cleaned for Swango, fell violently ill after he cooked a meal for her, her nephew recalled for investigators. He reported she was sweating, vomiting, and complaining of severe heartburn. He did not know it, but the nephew was describing the symptoms suffered by the Quincy paramedics. That night, Edith was rushed to an emergency clinic. By morning, she was dead.

Another suspected victim was the foreman of the hospital. He died while recovering from a leg amputation soon after being examined by Swango. So did a woman being treated after a miscarriage.

Then, one night, a woman in the maternity ward began screaming for help after seeing Swango inject something into her intravenous drip. She broke into a sweat and vomited but survived to deliver a healthy baby.

Finally, the hospital acted and called in the police. Hospital brass admitted to a local reporter that they tried to keep all their suspicions about Swango under wraps because they desperately needed a skilled doctor.

The police investigation discovered fifty-five different drugs in Swango's apartment. When questioned, he arrogantly responded that he came to the jungle out of the goodness of his heart and brought his own drugs. Swango was dismissed from the Mnene facility.

Back in Bulawayo, Swango rented a room in the home of a woman named Lynette O'Haire, a prominent socialite. Within a few weeks of having Swango as a border she began to have the same symptoms that other victims of the madman suffered. She had bouts of nausea, vomiting, severe headaches, and diarrhea.

O'Haire visited Doctor Michael Cotton, who worked at the same hospital as Swango and was a strong supporter of the American. But after examining O'Haire the doctor suspected arsenic poisoning. He sent hair samples to Pretoria, South Africa, for forensic analysis. The lab reports were sent to the Zimbabwe police, who shared them with Interpol, who sent them on to the FBI. Swango was called in for questioning by the Zimbabwe Criminal Investigations Department but they were not equipped to nail him down and he was released. However, once again he felt a noose tightening around his neck and fled, first to Zambia and then to Namibia, where he was hired for some medical work. We all found this impossible to believe.

The Zimbabwe government was determined to not let him get away with murder and they charged him *in absentia* with the poisonings.

In March 1997, Swango applied for a position at a hospital in Dhahran, Saudi Arabia. That was where he was headed when he was captured at O'Hare and held on the fraud charges.

Back in the States, my team reported that, judging from interviews, records, and anecdotal evidence, it was entirely possible that Swango killed as many as sixty patients during his approximately three years in Africa. The FBI agreed with the conclusion but Tom and Samantha, who interviewed many of the staff members in Mnene and Mpilo, thought the figure could be even higher. Swango now became an international MSK.

So, as I had hoped when I first met with Cecilia Gardner, the day she advised me not to work with Doctor Baden,

Swango was in jail for fraud and his time there turned out to be the most productive. From Quincy, Illinois, to Sioux Falls, North Dakota, to Newport News, Virginia, to Northport, New York, and on to Zimbabwe, Zambia, and Namibia, we traced a trail of suspicion, horror, disgust, and death that by all accounts could lead to one hundred innocent victims of an MSK. I feel to this day that if the FBI did not totally ignore me at that first meeting after Stony Brook, we may have stopped Swango before he went to Africa. That would have saved at least sixty lives.

Now, all that remained was to get a jury to believe us. It was legal crunch time. When AUSA Gary Brown called to alert me that Swango was almost due to be released on his fraud charge, I told him we were ready to present what we had in terms of a murder indictment. I remember Swango's own attorney commenting that she was also afraid of Swango getting out and being free to kill again.

Tom told me he wanted to contact the Zimbabwe government directly to inform them that Swango could possibly be out of prison soon. He thought they should file charges and request his extradition based on their charge he poisoned patients.

That was an extraordinary move because under usual circumstances, federal agents are not allowed to contact a foreign government without going through the State Department. However, we were dealing with a serial killer and up until now our level of cooperation from other agencies was almost nil. I told Tom to go ahead while I called the State Department. Shortly after, I received notice that Zimbabwe had filed indictments charging Swango with poisoning seven patients, including killing five of them. Subsequently, they contacted the State Department and requested extradition.

On July 11, 2000, the feds filed a criminal complaint charging Swango with three counts of murder, one count of assault, and one count each of false statements, mail fraud, and conspiracy to commit fraud. One week later, he was formally indicted and pleaded not guilty.

Following that, AUSA Gary Brown, and Swango's lawyer visited Swango in the Metropolitan Correctional Center in Manhattan where he was being held. It was revealed to him that our investigators had been to Africa and that Zimbabwe had filed charges against him that included murder. They told him there was an outcry in Africa to have him arrested and executed there.

He was offered a deal of changing his plea to guilty and accepting a life sentence by which he would avoid extradition to Zimbabwe. He took the deal.

Surprisingly, Swango was not a tough nut to crack. Psychiatrists who examined him before his sentencing reported he was fascinated by death. His father used to tell him war stories about killing men and how they died. He admitted sitting in a patient's room after administering a lethal injection and watching him die. He felt no compassion for the victims or their families. He just seemed to enjoy being intimate with death.

On September 6, 2000, Swango, wearing a blue prison jumpsuit and slippers, stood straight as a Marine and an honor guard before Judge Jacob Mishler in U.S. District Court in Central Islip, NY, to answer for his crimes. Before making his confession required by his plea deal, which spared him the death penalty, Swango and the audience in the courtroom—which contained families of his victims—had to endure the official record delivered by prosecutors.

Swango, now forty-five years old, stood as Assistant U.S. Attorney Gary Brown read five scrawled pages from the killer's diary that was seized from him when he was arrested in Chicago. The diary indicated Swango devoured books about doctors who killed their patients. I wondered if that diary was the reason Swango would not let me search his room at Northport. He must have been afraid I would find it. Alone it proved nothing, but with all the other circumstantial evidence, it painted him as a cruel, sadistic killer who loved to watch people die.

From one book on his reading list he copied in his diary: "He could look at himself in a mirror and tell himself that he was one of the most powerful and dangerous men in the world—he could feel that he was a god in disguise."

From another he copied: "When I kill someone it is because I want to. It's the only way I have of reminding myself that I am still alive," and then the words that seem to explain Michael Swango best: "I love it. Sweet, husky, close smell of an indoor homicide."

When Swango got his turn to address the court, his words chilled the large courtroom.

Without hesitation and in a loud voice easily heard in the farthest seat in the gallery, Swango said he intentionally went to Northport on his day off and murdered George Siano. One nurse told me she saw Swango sitting near the veteran's bed watching him slip away.

On other days he killed Aldo Serini and Thomas Sammarco while they were also patients at Northport Veterans Administration Medical Center.

Almost proudly, he explained to the judge how he used epinephrine and a paralyzing drug to kill his patients. "I did this by administering a toxic substance, which I knew was likely to cause death. I knew what I did was wrong."

He also pleaded guilty to two fraud counts, which included an admission he murdered the gymnast Cynthia McGee in Ohio, injected toxins into another veteran in Northport who survived, and poisoned two patients at a mission hospital in Zimbabwe.

Before Judge Mishler announced his sentence, the families of victims were given the opportunity to speak.

"He's worse than an animal. Animals don't kill for pleasure," said Siano's stepdaughter, Roselinda Conroy.

Sammarco's daughter, Carol Fisher, in tears, told the judge, "I hope he rots in hell."

Kristin Kinney's parents kept in touch with us for seven years since their daughter took her own life. We had the hair they took from her body just before cremation. It was found to be loaded with arsenic. Doctor Baden reasoned Swango had been feeding it in small doses to his fiancée.

The judge agreed to read a victim's statement from the parents of Kristin Kinney even though Swango was not charged in her death. Everyone in the room believed he was responsible for her suicide. The note read as follows:

> My daughter, Kristin Lynn Kinney, was engaged to be married to Doctor Michael Swango. However, on July 15, 1993 we were told that she had taken her own life. It is my belief and that of my husband's that Doctor Swango had a hand in her death. When we saved a tress of Kristen's hair on the day of her viewing, we had no idea that it would lead us on such a long and horrible seven-year journey to discover what really happened to Kristen.

Thanks to the efforts of Mr. Tom Valery of the Veterans Administration, a sample of that hair was tested for poison and was found to contain a toxic material. It is our belief that this toxic material strongly affected my daughter's judgment and mental orientation on the day of her death. According to a therapist, who saw her just before she died, she was incoherent, screaming and crying uncontrollably.

My husband (Al Cooper) and I, as well as the remainder of Kristin's family, respectfully request that the above information be weighed by you in any decisions you may make concerning the pleas made by Doctor Swango in respect to all of the charges that have been filed against him.

I have struggled not only with the death of my daughter, but with the fact that as a Registered Nurse and member of the Medical Profession, I am responsible for the welfare of the sick. Many years ago I took an oath that I would do my best, as a nurse, to protect those who are ill and in my care. It was with that in mind that I could not walk away suspecting there was a doctor killing people. After working with the FBI and Tom Valery of the Inspector General's Office of the VA for the past seven years, I hope that I have upheld my oath and that his knowledge will encourage the public to believe that there are many of us who cherish life and fight to save it.

Respectfully yours,

Sharon Cooper, RN

Everyone in the courtroom sat completely still, as quiet as possible, as Judge Mishler announced the sentence.

Swango was sentenced to three consecutive life terms without the possibility of parole. The judge made the unusual pronouncement that even though he was sentencing Swango to life without the possibility of parole, if Congress should change the law and allow Swango to seek parole, his request for parole is denied in advance. I had never heard that before or since.

Looking across the room at Swango I thought of that day in the tiny room at Northport. I remembered his arrogance, his defiance, and my impression that he would make a good match for my daughter. While he stood ramrod straight behind the defense table as Judge Mishler read the law, I could see he was drained. He had just served almost three years in prison and was now facing the rest of his life behind bars. He was a beaten man. I noticed a scar on his face I had not noticed before. I wondered if some jailhouse justice had been handed out. I had no compassion for him.

As the sentence was being read, I was shocked to see one of Swango's attorneys patting him on the back as if to console a poor victim. I turned away in disgust.

As of this writing, Swango is a sixty-three-year-old inmate at the nation's toughest prison, Supermax, in Florence, Colorado. I am sure he has no curtain to hide behind.

CHAPTER 9

Gilbert

"It would not be possible to praise nurses too highly."
—STEPHEN AMBROSE

While Swango was on the run, word was spreading around the VA that I was on to something not usually pursued by IG offices; but no one interfered, especially with nothing pressing on the case at the time. I thought it was good for the reputation of my office that we be involved in something challenging that was still up in the air regarding a final outcome.

It was a good time for me to clear my desk of other work and give Tom a break as well. I thought about a vacation for Eileen and me. Maybe a cruise somewhere. That was an idea put in my mind, since I arrested seventy-eight-year-old ID thief Rose Diamond while Swango was on the run.

A bank in the Bronx alerted my office that someone had been forging the name of a deceased widow of a veteran in order to steal her benefit checks. The widow, Mollie Diamond, died in 1970, so the scheme had been going on for more than twenty years. I took a trip up to the bank and quickly learned that the checks were being deposited in the joint account of the widow, Mollie, the rightful beneficiary, and her daughter, Rose.

At first, I could not understand why the bank would not have challenged Rose. I figured she must have had a good sob story, like she was a single mother with four kids and needed the money to survive. But the tellers, when I questioned them, insisted that Mollie was coming in to cash the checks. But I knew Mollie was deceased.

Leaving the bank, I went a few blocks away to Mollie's last known address, in a decrepit prewar building. An old woman with the appearance of a too common New York street character called a "bag lady" opened the door, looked at my ID card, and welcomed me into her living room. She said she was Mollie's daughter, Rose and that Mollie had died years earlier.

Without hesitation, she gave herself up and explained how she told the bank tellers that Mollie was sick at home and could not come in to cash the checks herself. Then using Mollie's Social Security number and her own photo ID, she opened an account at another bank, so she would have a place to keep the money and withdraw it when she needed it. The VA forensic accountants said she scammed at least seventy-five thousand dollars.

I was astounded that this seemingly helpless woman cooked up and carried out such a scheme. Looking around the apartment's ancient worn furnishings and meager decorations, I asked her what she did with the money.

"Did you ever go on a cruise, agent?" she said in response to my question.

I told her I had not but that my wife and I talked about it often.

"Oh, you are really missing out on a great experience. You should do it," she said.

Then she went on to describe the cruises she took all over the world—Greece, Spain, England, the Caribbean Islands, and Israel—all at the expense of US taxpayers, with money intended only to care for the widow of a World War II veteran. She went on and on and I admit I was an ardent listener. She told me how to get the best travel deals, which cruise lines to avoid, and the best times of the year to visit certain places.

In 1982, she spent the Christmas holidays in Hawaii, again courtesy of the Department of Veterans Affairs. In all, she spent about fifty thousand dollars on her trips.

She was quite a character and after rolling around in the slime with the Swango crowd for three years, I could not help but feel a soft spot for this lonely woman who found a way to bring joy to her life. In her mind, of course, she hurt no one. But I saw that differently. She took what was not hers to take. I do admit to thinking her father, the deceased vet, would probably have wanted her to have the money. He might be angrier towards me for putting a stop to it than at her for stealing. But it never entered my mind to shirk my duty.

This next part was somewhat embarrassing. I got a warrant to arrest Rose and a few days later, went up to the Bronx to collect her and bring her to the prisoner processing center for the Southern District of New York. The place was run by the US Marshals and they are a no-nonsense bunch who handle the worst of the worst, like Mafia hit men, bank robbers, and terrorists. They insist that any prisoner being brought into the facility be handcuffed behind his or her back.

Imagine the looks I got as I, along with another agent and a postal inspector who was involved in the investigation, paraded Rose through the building. Along the way, we ran into an FBI agent I knew who was escorting two hulking, sinister-looking characters. I asked him what they were being processed for.

Looking at my small group surrounding tiny handcuffed Rose, the agent smirked and said, "These two guys stuck up a bank and escaped with four thousand dollars. I've been hunting them for months."

"Oh yeah," I said, "Well, Rose, here, beat the U.S. Government out of seventy-five thousand dollars!"

At that, the two bank robbers laughingly cheered Rose, saying, "Right on mama, right on!"

When the marshals came to take her to another area to be processed, she got a standing ovation and wolf whistles from the collection of mopes crowded into the holding area. I wish I could have been inside when she delivered her lecture on the joys of cruising to the hard-nosed marshals.

Things turned out okay for Rose. She eventually pleaded guilty, got six months' probation, and did not have to pay back the money. I figured that left her with twenty-five thousand dollars' worth of cruises on the government still in the bank. I hope her father is smiling down on that.

Since the completion of that investigation, the VA routinely matches the names and Social Security numbers of its benefit recipients with the Social Security death listings. However, I know for a fact that there are still ID thieves who try to get away with the same scam.

Not long after, Eileen and I took a wonderful cruise to Bermuda, which I paid for myself. When I returned, a nurse named Kristen Gilbert quickly sucked me back into the quicksand world of MSKs.

I first heard her name during the winter of 1996, while Swango was on the run in Africa. Three nurses, John Wall,

Katherine Rix, and Renee Walsh, who worked at the Veterans Administration Medical Center in Northampton, Massachusetts, made allegations to management against a highly proficient nurse named Kristen Gilbert. The nurses were alarmed that the death rate on Gilbert's shift of patients in Ward C, which housed chronically ill patients and the Intensive Care Unit, was exceptionally high and thought an increase in the procurement of epinephrine might be somehow connected to that. Behind her back they began calling Gilbert the "Angel of Death." She looked like an angel, but she delivered death to patients who otherwise should have recovered. The nurses thought the circumstances of their deaths should be investigated.

The hospital administration listened to the trio of whistleblowers and called in Washington. But their attitude remained that doctors and nurses do not kill their patients. No amount of evidence would change their attitude.

Because of their persistence, a team from the VA Office of Healthcare Inspections traveled up to Northampton to look into the allegations and go over the records of the deceased in question.

The healthcare team did its work as trained to do and returned a report that agreed the death rates went up when Gilbert was present, and that these were unexpected deaths. Many occurred during code emergencies; that is, sudden attacks that could lead to death for one reason or another. But all the healthcare team was trained to do was ensure that the proper medical procedures were followed. It determined that procedures were followed, and that Gilbert showed exceptional ability in response to codes. It was not their job to look for possible criminality, which frustrated the three nurses who believed Gilbert was somehow responsible.

The team's report was circulated among VA brass in Washington and my boss, fully aware of my ongoing work on Swango, thought it would be a good idea for me to take a criminal investigator's look at the Northampton matter. He passed the Gilbert case to me and arranged a briefing by the healthcare team.

After my initial review, I saw missing epinephrine and identified Gilbert's proficiency at code responses as red flags, similar to Swango's MO. Also troubling was the fact that Gilbert worked the midnight shift, when she would be pretty much alone on the ward. That was another red flag. Those circumstances matched closely with what we had learned about Swango.

So, I dispatched Agent Jeff Hughes from my New Jersey office to lead a small team up to Northampton to interview the three nurses and other staff that had already been interviewed by the team. The difference would be that this time, they would be looking at the anecdotal and written evidence from a cop's point of view. The team's arrival set off a barrage of phone calls to DC from the Northampton administrators complaining that the agents were a distraction and there was nothing amiss at their facility. My bosses backed my aggressive move. That indicated a positive change in DC to me. Shoddy work and half-assed supervision would no longer be overlooked in favor of maintaining the VA's image.

Gilbert was not the first VA nurse to be labeled the "Angel of Death." Long before I became involved in suspicious-death investigations, a nurse struck terror at a VA Medical Center in the Midwest. From 1975 to 1985, VA nurse Donald Harvey murdered at least fifteen patients while working at the Cincinnati VA Medical Center. Remarkably, Harvey had been an inpatient at the VA Medical

Center in Lexington, Kentucky, for psychological reasons before he was ever hired as a VA nurse. He had been given electric shock treatments by the VA to control his inner demons, and was eventually released against the advice of his mother, who complained that her son was still as crazy as ever. Unbelievably, despite this medical history, he was given employment at the VA Medical Center in Cincinnati as a nurse. He didn't even have to forge résumés or government documents, as Swango had done to convince Stony Brook University to hire him.

Many years later, it was discovered that Harvey kept a rather precise diary on how he killed patients under his care. Sometimes he would press a plastic bag and wet towel over the mouth and nose of victims, or he would sprinkle rat poison in a patient's dessert. Other times, he would add arsenic or cyanide to their food or feeding tube, or inject them directly in the buttocks. Harvey eventually left the VA and began work at a private hospital, where he came under suspicion and his diary of death was uncovered. At various times and in various court rooms in 1987 and 1988, Harvey pleaded guilty to a total of approximately forty counts of murder throughout Ohio and Kentucky. Eighteen of his victims were veterans. He pleaded guilty and was sentenced to life without parole.

In 1978, he told a judge, "I felt what I was doing was right. I was putting people out of their misery. I hope if I'm ever sick and full of tubes or on a respirator, someone will come and end it."

Well, his life did not end the way he had hoped. On March 17, 2017, he was attacked in his cell at the Toledo Ohio Correctional Institute by another inmate. He died two days later.

"He's no mercy killer," said Arthur M. Ney Jr., the Ohio prosecutor who handled his case. "He killed because he liked to kill."

When my team returned to New York, Agent Hughes gathered them in a conference room and called me in. He filled me in on what they had heard from the Northampton staff about nurse Gilbert and what little they could glean from a few records that were made available to them by the reluctant administrators. The undeniable fact was that when this nurse was on duty in Ward C, patients died unexpectedly. When she was off duty, the death rate on the ward dropped to normal rates. Statistically, the probability of her being at the scene of all these suspicious deaths was next to impossible. Something we suspected about Swango was that the patients who died on his watch were almost always on their way to recovery. The same appeared to be true with Gilbert.

One anecdote they passed on to me was particularly chilling. It was about the day Gilbert was on duty in the ICU and got a call from her boyfriend, who was a police officer on the Northampton VA Medical Center, much like my friend Hank Shemitz at Northport, where Swango did his dirty work. Gilbert told her supervisor that her boyfriend had dinner reservations and asked if she could leave early that day.

The supervisor denied her request. He told her that ICU nurses were expected to stay with their patients until their conditions changed enough for them to be removed to regular wards. She noted that Gilbert's patient was on the road to recovery. She told Gilbert to check in later if the condition improved.

About two hours later, Gilbert returned to the supervisor to report that the patient had passed away. The supervisor was surprised but did not suspect wrongdoing. Gilbert was able to make it to the special dinner with her boyfriend.

When questioned by Hughes, the supervisor realized that the unexpected death of a patient should have set off alarms and called for a forensic investigation, but that was never done at Northampton. She too thought Gilbert was the "Angel of Death." But to call her a murderer would take more than anecdotal or circumstantial evidence.

Hughes' team picked up a lot of background information on what was going on in Gilbert's life at the time. They learned that during the summer of 1995, she began an affair with James Perrault, a medical center police officer who worked the same hours as she. At the time she was married to Glenn Gilbert, whom she met when she was a student at Greenfield Community College in Massachusetts and he was enrolled in a nearby college. In January 1988, they eloped. They had two young children when she began her affair with Perrault.

When a patient codes, Northampton rules required that a hospital police officer respond to the code location. Because they worked the same shift, when a Ward C patient coded, she and Perrault would both be on the scene, especially when she was the one who called in the code. One nurse said that when Perrault was present, Gilbert would always get as close as possible to him and the two would "play footsie," as the polite nurse put it. One witness recalled a code when Gilbert straddled a patient while performing CPR and brazenly showed off a new set of garters to Perrault.

These were the kinds of reports made by the three nurses who complained to their supervisors and were initially ignored.

During the investigation, Hughes also learned on Valentine's Day 1993, Gilbert called police saying she received a bomb threat over the phone. The caller said a bomb would explode in Ward C very shortly. Staff from throughout the hospital was called to Ward C to help evacuate its patients, including those in ICU. Police commanders were suspicious from the start because Ward C had been the site of several small fires, set over the past year, that added up to nothing but nuisance calls for the fire department, but caused commotion in the wards. They suspected an inside job.

Their suspicions increased when Gilbert found the "bomb" in an IV closet. It was made up of a Kleenex box attached to a small bag of IV fluid wrapped in tape. The cops remembered that she also was on duty when the fires were reported, and she was the one who located them.

One of her friends told the police that Gilbert once had to take a polygraph test following a suspicious fire in a nursing home where she worked.

When he finished debriefing me and the rest of the team, Hughes asked the six investigators in the room who had participated in the interviews to raise their hands if they thought Gilbert was guilty of murdering patients. All six raised their hands.

Everything I heard convinced me I would need a crackerjack team of investigators on the ground in Northampton. Tom Valery had a couple of other serious local cases and I wanted him in New York just in case there was a development in Swango. So he was not available. That would be a loss.

Fortuitously, when the nurses complained to Washington, they informed the local OIG of their concerns. That office assigned an expert agent to quietly take a look at what might be going on. His name was Steve Plante and I knew him by reputation. He was an 1811 investigator and I decided to add him to the team.

An 1811 is a civil service ranking that is extremely coveted and therefore, difficult to achieve. The 1811 must be a college graduate and complete the intensive criminal investigator training program at the Federal Law Enforcement Training Center in Glynco, Georgia. It is intended to prepare an investigator to tackle just about any crime imaginable, from kiddie porn to terrorism.

Once they complete that course, special agents of the Office of Inspectors General are required to attend IG Basic School for three weeks. To a large extent, the training is geared toward the investigation and prosecution of white-collar criminals, simply because most of the crimes investigated by the OIGs until Swango were financial in nature.

Plante was legendary in the VA for submerging himself in a case for weeks, months, or even years, and emerging with a conviction. He was known as a traveling agent or an agent who moved around the country wherever the case took him.

Each 1811 had his/her own style of investigating. Some were very successful at using the Colombo method; others were equally successful coming across as real tough guys. Most people who had dealt with Plante on a professional basis described him as an investigator who was very professional in appearance and demeanor, and sympathetic to the concerns of his witnesses and sources. People initially reluctant to speak to an investigator soon become comfortable in Plante's presence and begin to reveal their stories. Plante understood that I would be splitting my time between Northampton and my Special Agent in Charge duties in New York and that Hughes had a full plate in New Jersey. So, he realized early on that this matter was simply too complex for one investigator on the ground to handle alone. In short order, I put together one of the best investigative teams with whom I ever had the honor of working. It included Trooper Kevin Murphy, a homicide detective from the Massachusetts State Police.

Murphy looked the part. He was tall, serious, and, most importantly, extremely knowledgeable about his craft, the investigation of murder. Murphy had worked homicide cases for more than twenty years. What impressed me most was his thorough understanding of medical terminology, and his familiarity with the processes of exhumation and autopsy that he had witnessed on hundreds of occasions. I knew Doctor Baden, who I fully intended to bring on board, would appreciate Murphy as a consummate professional.

Having a state police homicide investigator and pairing him with an 1811 of Plante's caliber was an extraordinary opportunity to do great police work.

The Gilbert team had all the elements that were necessary for a successful team operation. Over a very short period, a tremendous camaraderie developed among our members. Most important, however, each team player gave 110 percent effort. This team, which accomplished the near impossible, should be viewed as a model for law enforcement teamwork everywhere.

As Spring 1996 arrived, it was time for me to get up to Northampton to meet with Assistant US Attorney William Welch. I was quite impressed by the town of North Hampton. It reminded me of a combination of Greenwich Village and Southampton on Long Island rolled into one. Smith College is located there. The downtown atmosphere is artsy and touristy.

The VA medical center was in the woodsy Leeds section of town on a 105-acre area called Bear Hill. Like other VA facilities in suburban areas, the property was well cared for and offered a calming, healing, almost country club atmosphere.

Its more than two dozen small red brick buildings contained 191 beds, and the winding roadways around the property brushed up against several attractive fountains. It dated back to 1922, when President Warren G. Harding signed legislation that led to the clearing of Bear Hill of its distinctive pine trees and the building of the medical center. It was the VA's first psychiatric medical center, and in those days, cared for many WWI veterans.

I had visited dozens of VA facilities in my career and Northampton was typical of the institutional look and feel of the 1930s' style of VA medical center care. Only limited surgical services were offered there. Seriously ill patients were often transferred to more sophisticated medical centers.

It was extremely difficult to recruit and retain doctors and nurses for those types of facilities. The pay was generally not as lucrative as that offered by the private sector, and the in-patients in Gilbert's day were mostly acute, long-term care patients who suffered from numerous long-term ailments. Consequently, a percentage of the staff was only employed on a part-time basis. Such was the case with registered nurse Kristen Gilbert, who started there March 6, 1989, assigned to the main medical unit in Building One. At that time, the entire facility was almost two hundred beds spread over twenty-six buildings. These days, it has about fifty beds concentrating on psychiatric issues.

Remembering my contretemps with Loretta Lynch, I did not look forward to the meeting with AUSA Welch. I took Plante with me. With fingers crossed, I entered Welch's office praying my reception would be more welcoming than I ever got from Lynch and the Eastern District of New York. I knew that every day, federal prosecutors are referred cases from a host of federal agencies. A virtual alphabet soup of agencies is at their door clamoring for attention, like the FBI, DEA, OIG, Immigration and Customs Enforcement (ICE), Defense Criminal Investigative Service (DCIS), Naval Criminal Investigative Service (NCIS), and so on. and on. They obviously can't accept all their cases, so they must have a method with which to pick and choose.

Often knowing the agent referring the case can make all the difference. If they have worked with him/her before, and have confidence in his/her abilities, they may be more inclined to accept a case from that person rather than a stranger. It's only natural.

Welch was the federal prosecutor for Springfield, Massachusetts. He had never met Plante or me, and we were from an agency with whom he had never worked. And now we were asking the prosecutors to assist in the investigation and prosecution of a professional caregiver at the local VA hospital who may have murdered her patients. We had no eyewitness, no motive, no weapon, and no forensic evidence to convince them. There was only anecdotal evidence that when this nurse was on duty, people died unexpectedly. And to make matters worse, there had already been reviews concluding hospital procedures were followed correctly by VA healthcare inspectors. Any prosecutor knew that an endeavor like this could take years to complete and might not result in a favorable outcome. The FBI tried to make a case like this before in Columbia, Missouri, in 1992 and failed after a valiant effort that cost the Bureau dearly in time, money, and adverse publicity. As a result, they declined to get involved in the Gilbert matter. However, that was the best news I had heard.

Welch was a godsend, a total professional crime fighter. He was much more willing to push the envelope than the attorneys in the Eastern District of New York. We told him about our suspicions regarding Gilbert and filled him in on the Swango case. He asked me a few good questions. I told him what we were learning about the telltale signs a killer doctor may be at work. The signs included the unexpected deaths of patients on the way to recovery, the interest and proficiency at code emergencies, and of course, the missing epinephrine, which we had learned could serve a deadly purpose and be almost impossible to detect in a body after death. He said he would be the lead prosecutor and that he would bring in Assistant U.S. Attorney Ariane Vuono, a former state prosecutor with experience in homicide investigations. This was a great team and ready to go.

Welch soon secured two search warrants, one for Gilbert's home, which she had shared with her husband and two little boys up until recently when they separated; the other one was for her apartment, where she was said to be shacking up with her boyfriend, James Perrault, the Northampton VA cop. These warrants allowed us to show up unannounced, a big advantage when there was suspected evidence that could be destroyed like epinephrine, which could be flushed down a toilet as we waited in the hallway for someone to open the door and let us in.

Warrants like this are very intimidating. They display the full power and force of the US government. Welch was also pleased we had a Massachusetts State Police officer aboard in case the eventual facts of the crime failed to rise to federal standards. There is no murder statute on the federal books unless the murder is committed on a federal reservation such as a military base or a VA medical center. We needed to prepare for any eventuality, including trying the case in state court.

I understood I was miles ahead of where we were when we grilled Swango in the small room at Northport. I had the results from Hughes and his team. We had total cooperation from the nurses in Ward C and we had the US Attorney totally aboard. After the meeting, I returned to New York.

After a few days back in New York, I took the ferry from Port Jefferson, Long Island, not far from my home across the Long Island Sound, to Connecticut, then drove up to Northampton.

I enjoyed the ferry trip. It was very relaxing, like a sea cruise, and it gave me a feeling of really going somewhere far away. Occasionally the Long Island Sound could be rough and on one trip, I stood on an upper deck and watched as my government car took a beating from waves and hard rain down below me. I thought for a moment it would get washed away. I had a quick thought about having to restore it in my garage before my boss found out. It would have been a challenge.

CHAPTER 10

Detectives at Work

*"A detective sees death in all the various forms
at least five times a week."*

—EVAN HUNTER

I decided to hit Gilbert's former home first. I took Steve Plante along and without prior notice, we politely knocked on her husband Glenn Gilbert's door early one morning. Executing a warrant is always a tense situation no matter what you are looking for. The suspect is often nervous and fearful, and we had to be alert to any sudden movements and attempts to hide damaging evidence.

Glenn was relaxed when he opened the door and led us into the living room. He sat on the sofa and we sat across from him on two comfortable chairs. The kids were in school. We showed him the warrants and explained that we wanted to talk about his relationship with Kristen, and then we wanted to look through the house for certain items she may have kept there. We told him he could make our job easier if he knew of any drugs or medical instruments, like syringes or literature relating to drugs or poisons, she may have left there when she moved out. He said he did not believe we would find anything like that.

We asked him about any strange behavior he may have noticed over the past few years. He candidly told us he knew about her affair with Perrault and that friends told him she had been sneaking off from work to meet with him. He knew she told their mutual friends that she was thinking of leaving her husband. She went on a strict diet and changed her hairstyle. He noticed she bought new perfume and lingerie. Northampton was a small town and there were few things that stayed secret. Glenn said he was told by one of Kristen's coworkers that she was wearing sexy lingerie beneath her nurse's uniform and showing it off to female friends. Glenn confirmed what we already knew—that Kristen had resigned from the hospital.

After a few minutes, we did our search of the small house, going through kitchen cabinets, bathroom medicine chests, hall closets, and chests in the bedrooms. We even looked in the boys' room. It is a very intimate process. We were seeing private objects not usually meant to be seen. But we found nothing incriminating.

We left Glenn and decided to go straight to Kristen's apartment. Plante said he had already heard a lot of that kind of gossip about Kristen but we let Glenn talk hoping we would pick up a tiny bit of new information that could lead to something else. Kristen's fling with Perrault did not indicate she was murdering patients.

I began wondering just how much a part Perrault might have played in whatever evil Gilbert was doing. *Could we have two MSKs working in partnership?*

Plante, Murphy, and I met Kristin Gilbert for the first time when we arrived at her apartment. We were surprised to find the door open and she and Perrault sitting in the living room.

My first impression was of her physical appearance; she was certainly attractive, but in an icy-cold sort of way. She didn't attempt any pleasantries; she got right down to business, wanting to know what we were doing there. My vision of a serial killer, until I met Swango, had always been of a Charles Manson type, someone unkempt who looks crazy enough to kill. The vision of an attractive blonde nurse as a serial killer just didn't fit any profile I've ever harbored. But, by now, I knew better and nothing surprised me.

Perrault was an annoying jerk. Showing off for Gilbert, he started in questioning me as to whether we had a search warrant. Having previously been questioned by Hughes and Plante regarding this matter, he obviously knew what we were doing and was apparently just showing off for Gilbert. But I played his game, politely identifying myself and explaining that we had a search warrant in connection with an investigation of certain deaths at the Northampton Medical Center.

Failing to intimidate us, he shut his mouth and they both sat there as we did our work. All we found was a pharmacy book, but it interested me because the page on epinephrine was dog-eared. With the book in my hand, I approached Gilbert and asked her if she would like to talk about all the rumors buzzing around the hospital and town. And I wanted to ask her why she resigned from the hospital. While we were looking around, Gilbert called her lawyer.

All I got was that stone-cold stare in return. My thought was that I wouldn't want her caring for me if I were in Ward C. After a minute or two of more silence, Gilbert's lawyer walked in the door, identified himself, and said his client had nothing to say to us. He said if we were finished, we should leave. We were finished, so we left the apartment shortly thereafter. The next time I would see Gilbert would be at her trial.

Driving away from the apartment, I asked Plante if he thought Gilbert was a "code junkie." The anecdotal evidence he and Hughes were picking up indicated she was one of those medical staffers who enjoyed the rush of responding to an emergency and performing under great pressure. Swango, who had become my baseline reference point on investigating MSKs, loved code emergencies as well and often called them in himself. So now I was building a case comparing it to one that might never make it to court. That was not the best way to create a textbook on how to investigate MSKs, but it was taking shape in my mind and pointing me in the right directions.

Something that Murphy dug up at this time was really bothering me. In 1987, shortly after Gilbert graduated from nursing school, we learned that she took a job with the Visiting Nurse Association of Franklin County, Massachusetts. She disciplined a special needs child she was caring for by pouring scalding bathwater over his body. The child suffered severe burns over 60 percent of his body. Gilbert, as far as we could determine, was never disciplined for the incident and it apparently did not stand in the way of her future employment. I could only imagine that the nursing service was avoiding bad publicity by letting it go. Another pattern was forming in my mind. MSKs get away with many different forms of—to put it mildly—bad behavior before moving up to murder.

CHAPTER 11

Ward C

"Do you want to speak to the Doctor in charge,
or the Nurse who really knows what is going on?"

—UNKNOWN

I needed to take a look at Ward C. I wanted to get the feel
of the place to try to imagine Kristen Gilbert at work. My
presence in the hospital made everyone nervous so I waited
until the midnight shift, Gilbert's shift, when Ward C was
empty, to take my tour. It looked exactly like I had expected
it to, an old-style ward with rows of beds that were separated
by curtains, which I now instantly and unfairly referenced in
my mind as "murder curtains."

As I met with some of the staff, I sensed their mixed
feelings about this matter. On the one hand, they felt that
patients had died unexpectedly and Gilbert was somehow involved; yet on the other hand, they were hesitant to accuse a
coworker of intentionally murdering patients.

Not many people in my experience would actually come
forward to make allegations like that. I appreciated the

soul-searching that must have gone through the minds of the nurses before they made the decision to step up. Once the decision was made, they had better fasten their seat belts because they were in for the ride of their lives. Ostracism—from their coworkers and management, from other members of their profession, and even from members of their community or family—might leave them feeling they had placed their livelihoods in jeopardy. Putting all this aside, the three VA nurses—Wall, Rix, and Walsh—took just such a bold step. Their lives would never be the same.

"It was the most uncomfortable day of my life," said Wall. He told me how he brought his concerns before the head nurse, and then had to go back to the ward and assign Gilbert continuing patient care duties. He wanted to assign Gilbert to administrative duties while his supervisor wanted her to continue distributing medications. He had no choice but to allow her to pass out medications and during the entire evening that day, he could only think about Gilbert killing someone.

One afternoon, I received a call from Glenn Gilbert. He asked me to come to his house to search a pantry that was Kristen's personal territory when she lived there. Our search warrant was still in effect so Plante, Murphy, and I headed over as quickly as was we could.

Glenn pointed us to the pantry, which was packed with food cans and other items. On a back shelf, hidden from view, we found a book named the *Handbook of Poisoning*. The three of us looked at each other in amazement. Clearly, Glenn knew it was there, but we missed it on the first search. Glenn wanted us to have it. This sealed the deal for us. She was a killer, no doubt. We had to speed things up.

The following day Gilbert checked herself into a psychiatric hospital for the first time. She might have thought she could avoid us, but she was wrong.

This murder investigation was in full swing and Gilbert, now resigned from the hospital, was hanging around town speaking to everyone she knew about the "witch hunt" going on at Northampton. Her closest friends among the nurses were steering clear of her, afraid to get caught up in her madness.

She was aggressive about defending herself and returned to her old tricks. Gilbert knew that during early morning hours, Perrault would be answering the telephone at the hospital. She began making a series of threatening calls, including a bomb threat.

Perrault by now realized something was seriously wrong with his girlfriend and he tried to get her to stop calling. He ended their relationship, which only made her increase the calls, and they became more threatening. Up to this point, Perrault tried to take Gilbert's side in hospital water cooler talk and with local detectives and my team. He even expressed anger with her coworkers who cooperated with us but would not do so with Gilbert's lawyer and a private eye she hired. Her behavior indicated to me that there was much more to be uncovered about Gilbert than phony bomb threats and unnecessary code alerts. Perrault, realizing the same, agreed to cooperate with us.

One afternoon, Gilbert used her car to block Perrault's car in his driveway and pleaded with him not to keep an appointment with Plante and Murphy. She wailed that they were trying to frame her for things she had not done. Gilbert finally let him drive away but she followed him, and while he was inside speaking with the detectives, she vandalized his car.

During one session with Plante and Murphy, Perrault said that in a July 1996 phone call with her, she confessed to killing patients. When I heard this, I knew we had to step up the investigation. We needed to look at the records of deaths on Gilbert's watch, and then I would need my old friends Michael Baden and Fredric Rieders to come to Northampton.

The Northampton facility began to receive bomb threats. Kristen's now ex-boyfriend Perrault was on duty and answered the phone the day after we found the *Handbook of Poisoning*. The caller stated, "There are three explosives in Building One. You have two hours." The building, of course, had to be evacuated. Evacuating patients from an ICU is not an easy task. Not only is it logistically difficult, it obviously puts patients in harm's way. A total of fifty patients had to be evacuated.

Northampton police and the VA force responded. Perrault may have been foolish in choosing his girlfriends, but he was a pretty good cop. He told the first responders he could not recognize the caller's voice because he was convinced it was electronically altered. Before the evening was over, the VA medical center received twelve more threatening messages, and approximately twenty other messages from pay telephones over the course of the next several days. They all appeared to be made with the use of some voice-altering device. But the police techs did not believe it was a sophisticated device. They thought it was a toy.

Four days later, we were able to get a court order to have Gilbert placed in the Baystate Medical Center for psychiatric evaluation. This time it wasn't voluntary.

Plante was all over this. We all believed Gilbert had made the calls. Plante spoke to Gilbert's friends about her activities over the few days preceding the calls. He learned she had been shopping at the local mall before the calls were made.

Understanding he was looking for a toy, not something that would have been purchased at an electronics specialty store, he went to the town's Toys R Us first. There, with the cooperation of the store manager, he confirmed Gilbert purchased two voice-altering devices. The first was known as "Talkgirl Jr." The second, purchased days later, was a device known as "Talkboy Jr." They were toys for children to have fun with, but which we thought Gilbert had put to a sinister use.

Knowing Gilbert was in the psych ward at the time, Plante told me he wanted to go back to Gilbert's apartment to take a look around. I cautioned him not to try to go inside until we had a proper warrant. The facts that would prove Gilbert made those calls were beginning to pile up and I did not want anything to jeopardize that investigation. I thought of what was going on with the Swango team at the moment. We were using the time he was in prison on the fraud charge to build the murder charges against him. Maybe we could get Gilbert held on the bomb threat because that would give us time to pursue the murder case. I knew how time-consuming a murder investigation against an MSK could be. Exhumations, autopsies, and tissue analyses took time.

Plante went to Gilbert's apartment, where he fortuitously found the "Talkgirl Jr." in the bushes outside her front door. That was good news to us and the Northampton police, who wanted her for calling in the bomb threats. Murdering veterans was not yet on their radar.

I ordered a roving surveillance of Gilbert to go into action as soon as she left the psychiatric hospital. A week after my order, Baystate Medical Center accommodated us. A few minutes after she was on the street, we saw her making a telephone call from a phone booth approximately half a mile from her apartment. At the same time, Perrault received a call at his post in Northampton. He immediately alerted us to the call though he said he could only hear heavy breathing and traffic in the background. That was more than enough for us to get a new search warrant for Gilbert's home and by that afternoon we had the "Talkboy Jr." toy in an evidence bag.

The next day, Gilbert voluntarily returned to the psychiatric ward claiming she attempted suicide. We really could not touch her while she was in there under observation. But, two days later, when she checked herself out, she was arrested by Plante and Murphy, and soon after, indicted for making the bomb threats to the VA medical center.

After a week in jail, she was ordered to move to her parents' home in Setauket, Long Island, not far from my home, until her trial.

Her trial was the biggest thing to hit Northampton in decades. But it was not about murdering patients. Nevertheless, Plante, Murphy, and I sat through it with interest. We heard Perrault testify about his relationship with Gilbert as the prosecutor built his case that she was phoning in the threats to get the VA cop's attention. She was so obsessed with Perrault that he had to take a restraining order out against her. But because this was not a murder trial, the jury never heard about her confession that she killed a patient, the discovery of *Handbook of Poisoning*, the missing epinephrine, the increased death rate when she was on duty, and the nonsensical code alerts. Nevertheless, they heard enough to convict her for making false bomb threats to a federal institution. She was sentenced to fifteen months at Danbury Correctional Institution in Connecticut, where it was ordered she would receive psychiatric treatment.

To most people in town, she was just a harmless nutcase. Her friends and some of her colleagues saw her as a sad example of a very talented nurse whose inner demons destroyed a great career. Except for a few, they had no idea about her real inner demons. Plante, Murphy, and I knew her as a psychopathic killer and we were determined to prove it.

Gilbert's incarceration gave me the time I needed to concentrate on the real reason for my presence in Northampton, Plante's assignment, Murphy's involvement, and, of course, the bigger picture for the US Attorney's Office. We were now going to focus on Gilbert as a Medical Serial Killer. Anyone who doubted our theory now had to explain why, when not long after she was carted off to Danbury, the death rate in Ward C returned to normal, as did the epinephrine supply.

CHAPTER 12

Icing on the Cake

"The corpse is a silent witness who never lies."

—ANONYMOUS

U p to now, the Gilbert team had all the elements of a
successful operation. Every member was a team player
and gave 100 percent of themselves to the effort. My office,
the US Attorney's Office, the Massachusetts State Police, the
Northampton Police, and the police at Northampton VA
Medical Center worked hand in hand in pursuit of Kristen
Gilbert, and she was in Danbury Federal Correctional Institution as a result. But we all knew that was not why we originally joined forces. And now we needed to expand our team.

It was time for the brainiacs, my good friends Drs. Michael Baden and Fredric Rieders, and a brilliant cardiologist
they knew at VA Medical Center in West Roxbury, Massachusetts, Doctor Thomas Rocco, to come aboard. They
would complement Bruce's Angels, who had proven their
worth on Swango.

The task at hand was to go through the Northampton records of the deceased patients identified as dying under questionable circumstances by the three nurses. They risked friendships and careers by coming forward to the VA with their suspicions about their colleague.

We would need to count those missing bottles of epinephrine, prove that Gilbert had access to them, prove they were administered to the patients in question, and finally, prove that they died from those injections. We had to be able to paint the picture for a jury that, given the opportunity and resources, Kristen Gilbert would draw the curtain around her patient, and for thrill and glory, administer a dose of fatal poison.

Doctor Rieders once told me that forensic science is just the icing on the cake. The cake itself is comprised of the actual investigation, the people, the witnesses, and the work of the street investigators. One should never rely on toxicology alone to make a case, as too many things can go wrong. Well, we were strong in that department. Plante and Murphy had seen to that and the more they dug, the more circumstantial evidence they turned up. But I knew we needed the scientists to bring it home to the jury even though it could be very complicated.

For instance, I had to picture Rieders on the witness stand. With his thick European accent and scientist-like appearance, he appeared to be a character right out of a science-fiction novel. Being on the cutting edge of forensic science, he was no stranger to controversy.

When you introduce new science never before utilized in a court of law, you better be prepared for the most grueling of challenges, both scientific and personal. Rieders was convinced he could find a byproduct of epinephrine, known as metanephrine, in embalmed, buried, and exhumed tissue. Normetanephrine is a metabolite of metanephrine that helps transmit nerve impulses. The ratio of metanephrine to normetanephrine in the tissue samples would be crucial because there would be more metanephrine only if the patients were injected with the drug. Rieders was convinced that his lab would find just such a ratio. He claimed that a new piece of equipment just recently set up in his office, known as the High Performance Liquid Chromatography Tatum Mass Spectrometry, would be able to find the byproducts of epinephrine.

It would be the job of Doctor Baden to bring the correct tissue to Rieders. His success rate was beyond challenge, and resulted in Swango's guilty plea. I am confident he was sent to prison forever by the work of Baden and Rieders.

Doctor Rocco's testimony would provide support that the veterans in question died of epinephrine poisoning—and not of natural causes or whatever they were being treated for at Northampton, when Gilbert got her hands on them in Ward C.

We intended to prove that on August 21, 1995, she killed Stanley Jagodowski, sixty-six, a Korean War vet who entered Northampton on July 21 with unbearable sores on his legs and feet. He had his right leg amputated just above the knee due to infection. He was overweight, had non-insulin dependent diabetes, and high blood pressure. He also had enlarged heart ventricles and an irregular heartbeat. Despite his many problems, he was recovering nicely when Gilbert killed him.

In 1985 another victim, Henry Hudon, thirty-five, an Air Force vet, suffered head injuries while breaking up a barroom brawl. He was struck in the back of his head and fell to the ground paralyzed. He had a detached retina and his front teeth shattered. He "recovered" from those injuries but was never the same. He was diagnosed with paranoid schizophrenia and was a frequent patient at Northampton because he fluctuated from "in control" to "out of control." In the fall of 1995, his condition worsened, and his doctors could not find the correct mixture of medications to help.

On December 7, 1995, Hudon was admitted to Northampton and sent to Ward C complaining of diarrhea and stomach problems. It was determined that he was lying about his condition and simply had the flu. Later that day, after being attended to by Gilbert, he went into cardiac arrest and died.

We thought she also killed Kenny Cutting, forty-one, on February 2, 1996, an Army vet who was diagnosed with multiple sclerosis. He was admitted to Northampton's long-term care program. While there, as his body deteriorated, he never lost his cheerfulness and was well-liked by the nurses and doctors. Eventually, after much testing, it was determined that Cutting did not have MS. He suffered from severe infections. After several procedures. he settled into a peaceful, relatively healthy situation.

On January 26, 1996, when he developed a high fever because of an infection, he was transferred to Ward C. Over the next several days he was attended to by Gilbert and other nurses. Working the night shift in a very quiet Ward C on February 2, 1996, Gilbert was told to report to ICU, where her only patient was Cutting. As previously stated, that evening she asked her supervisor for that shift, John Wall, if she could leave work early. Wall explained that in ICU, she needed to stay with the patient until there was some change in his condition. A few hours later, Gilbert killed Cutting and left work early.

It was shortly after she killed Cutting that the three heroic nurses came forward with their suspicions about their coworker.

Nevertheless, she continued her maniacal murderous mayhem.

Edward Skwira, sixty-nine, was a World War II Army vet. He was an alcoholic admitted to Northampton on February 15, 1996, for long-term care. He was in a state of mental confusion and had low blood pressure. In addition to his alcoholism, he suffered from hypertension, coronary artery disease, vascular disease, and carotid artery disease. Once Skwira was stabilized, he was sent to Ward C. That afternoon during her shift, Gilbert poisoned Skwira with epinephrine. By 6:30 that night, Skwira was transferred to another more specialized hospital, Baystate, to care for what doctors at Northampton thought was a severe heart issue. He never recovered from the poisoning and died two days later.

James Perrault's testimony to the grand jury about Gilbert's confession to killing patients in a phone call with him on July 10, 1996, eventually returned a murder indictment against her. Two days later, he took out a restraining order against her.

We also were certain she tried, but failed, to kill two other patients.

Angelo Vella, sixty-eight, a World War II Marine Corps hero was diagnosed with Chronic Obstructive Pulmonary Disease (COPD) and was admitted to Northampton's Ward C on February 4, 1996, with shortness of breath. After being stabilized during the day, Vella came under Gilbert's "care" that night. He was in no distress and was resting comfortably when Gilbert took over. Respiratory therapist Bonnie Bledsoe had administered treatment Vella's treatment and it was successful. Later that evening Gilbert injected Vella with epinephrine and it caused his heart monitor to go off. A code was called. There was a speedy response and Gilbert reluctantly helped save his life to the appreciation of everyone involved.

Thomas Callahan, sixty-one, a Korean War Army vet who also suffered from COPD, drank a bottle of whiskey a day and was schizophrenic. He was admitted to Northampton on January 18, 1996, with pneumonia. Four days later, Callahan was admitted to Ward C. In the hospital, he was detoxing and became violent. He had no problem with his heart. In fact, he was stable throughout the day. Later that evening, Callahan began to have heart issues because of an injection by Gilbert. After a code was called, Callahan was stabilized and saved by other doctors and nurses.

We identified the four dead patients that Baden should exhume for autopsies. We needed to get the families of the victims to cooperate. There was a lot of work ahead of us. We needed to compile records that followed the course of drug supplies, especially epinephrine; we needed to examine the results of code events involving Gilbert; and we needed to continue to collect all the anecdotal evidence that could be useful to prosecutors. But I had learned from Swango that the exhumation process—beginning with family approval, then court, then cemetery procedures—could eat up valuable time. In the Swango case, we had finished our work just under the gun, about a week before he was to be released from prison on the fraud charge. If we had missed that deadline, he might have once again found a way to disappear. I could not take that chance with Gilbert.

Fortunately, Plante developed an excellent relationship with the victim's families. He brought flowers to the gravesites and made certain that everything regarding our applications to the court and other preparations were done in a caring, professional manner. Plante's utmost professionalism was demonstrated when he made certain the victims' remains were returned to the gravesite as quickly as possible after the scientific analysis had been completed.

The exhumations went without a hitch. This time, I knew what to expect in terms of stench, "torture" instruments, and the overall atmosphere of death in the air. I was able to watch more intensely as the great Baden went about his work removing certain organs from the bodies, examining them in his hands while at the same time loudly describing what he was learning. The process was also preserved on a video recording as a medical record, concurrent with the actual actions of the examiner.

An autopsy is a very stressful event and like other stressful situations, humor is sometimes used to break the tension. During those moments, we were careful to turn off the audio system, as some off-the-cuff remarks would be made that could have had great impact on a jury. During the second Northampton autopsy, we neglected to shut down the audio during one of those tension-easing breaks. I was observing while Baden and Special Agent Brian Donnelly were doing the autopsy when Brian joked that maybe we should put some epi (epinephrine) in the body. It was only a joke to lighten up an intense situation. Unfortunately, the video and audio were going and this embarrassing joke had to be disclosed at trial, completely out of context to boot. It was embarrassing for all concerned and possibly put the entire case at risk. A lesson was definitely learned from the experience.

The exhumation and autopsy process continued for four months. When it concluded, a grand jury began hearing testimony from Perrault, Plante, Murphy, Glenn Gilbert, the three nurses, victim's families, hospital administrators, and then Doctors Baden and Rieders. On November 24, 1998, Kristen Gilbert was indicted for murdering the four veterans. She pleaded not guilty. She faced the death penalty.

In February of 1999, she was moved from her cell in Danbury to Hampden County Jail and House of Correction in Ludlow, Massachusetts, where she would await her trial.

Our case was simple yet complicated. The medical and technical elements would have to be explained to the jury in a way that would convince them that epinephrine could be a murder weapon. The jury would also need to be persuaded that a highly competent, educated, well-liked nurse could possess the mind of a merciless killer.

Simply put, Gilbert's MO began with the theft of epinephrine from Ward C's medicine cabinet. Then, when the ward was empty of other personnel, which was common during Gilbert's overnight shift, a shift she volunteered for, she would pull the bedside curtain around her. She would then inject the patient with a fatal dose of the drug. If she happened to be seen and questioned during this process, she would explain that she was flushing the patient's intravenous line with saline solution, an unusual and dangerous practice. Her victims all suffered from differing degrees of cardiac problems but were not expected to die.

Our argument was that by injecting the epinephrine into these particular patients, she was able to generate a medical emergency, a code, which she plausibly claimed was caused by a naturally occurring heart attack. Our theory, based on interviews with coworkers, her ex-husband Glenn Gilbert, and her lover, James Perrault, was that the codes brought her into contact with Perrault and the excitement and adrenalin rush she craved.

Her history with codes is one for the record books. As our investigation gathered more and more statistics matching up to her work, it was almost impossible to believe.

There were 106 deaths, sixty-three on Ward C/ICU where Gilbert was assigned. Of the sixty-three deaths, forty-four occurred on the evening shift, which she customarily worked. Of those forty-four deaths, Gilbert was on duty for thirty-seven. We eventually concluded she was on duty for 84 percent of the deaths that occurred on that ward. Gilbert found twenty-two of these deceased patients herself. The next nurse on the list of code patients found had a total of five in the same time frame. Add to those numbers the fact that the Northampton pharmacy delivered a staggering 115 ampules of epinephrine to Ward C during that period. Considering Gilbert was a part-time employee, working a thirty-two-hour a week shift, she was responsible for seventy-five codes. It appears she came to work just to kill patients.

When interviewing medical staff, I was never able to substantiate the claim of one staffer who told Plante she brought the unusual numbers to a supervisor who would not allege that a nurse was harming patients and chose to ignore her.

One male VA nurse told me that all the hospital personnel welcomed codes. He said, "When a code alert was sounded, it was a break from our regular, mundane work and an opportunity to use our skills to the highest degree. Nobody would deny it was an adrenaline rush and sometimes heroes emerged from the incident, often quick-thinking, highly competent nurses who otherwise toiled in obscurity." Over the years, I have heard that from many other hospital employees. It described Kristen to a tee. She was a glory hunter and had a desperate need for attention.

All this the jury would hear. We were building a very strong case against Gilbert. I could not be prouder of the dedicated detective work that was done by my investigators, the medical people, and, of course, the forensic nurses.

Yet, there was one story the court ruled the jury could not hear. It provided another glimpse into the bizarre world of Kristen Gilbert.

It occurred about a year before she began her intense affair with Perrault. At the time, Glenn Gilbert was hospitalized for gastroenteritis. We believed it was brought on by Gilbert, who administered low doses of diuretics in her husband's food over the preceding few weeks. It resulted in an unusually low level of potassium and glucose in his blood. Our medical experts said that would have explained his irregular heartbeat at the time. He was discharged from the hospital without follow-up tests. This was the first stage of an elaborate attempt by Gilbert to murder her husband.

Gilbert complained to her husband that he should not have been discharged without a blood test. The following day, she came home with two syringes, one of which was filled with a clear, odorless liquid. She told him she wanted to take a blood sample back to Northampton to have it checked for his potassium level. But first, she said, she had to inject him with saline solution to flush his vein.

Glenn told my team that as the injection went in his arms, his chest went numb. He tried to escape the needle, but his wife pinned him against a wall and continued the injection. Glenn briefly lost consciousness. He revived and survived without any further medical attention, especially from his wife.

Gilbert's explanation to Plante and homicide cop Murphy was that Glenn fainted at the sight of the syringe. Glenn did not report this attack until about five months after it occurred, when he and his wife were fighting over child custody. She was never indicted for it, but my team was convinced Gilbert was trying to induce a fatal heart attack in her husband, something she was adept at doing to at least four veterans at Northampton.

The court also ruled that the jury would not be allowed to hear about Gilbert's bomb threat conviction and the statistical claim that the chances of her being an attending nurse at so many deaths were one hundred million to one, which indicated she created the life or death situations.

But there was much more that they would hear.

CHAPTER 13

Trial of the Century

"It was a cold chilly day. On Ward C of the U.S.
Department of Veterans Affairs Medical Center, there
was a different kind of chill that penetrated the floor.
It was a deep eerie feeling; patients were dying
unexpectedly from sudden cardiac arrest. Three
nurses came together and voiced their suspicions.
It was every hospital's nightmare. There was a killer
among them, one who coldly and callously killed
four men and attempted to kill two others by injecting
them with the heart stimulant epinephrine..."

—ASSISTANT U S ATTORNEY WILLIAM WELCH II
Opening remarks of the trial of Kristen Gilbert, November
2001

For Northampton, this would be the trial of the century.
Kristen Gilbert faced the death penalty even though it was
abolished in the Commonwealth of Massachusetts in 1984.
The last State execution was in 1947, when two men were
electrocuted for murder. The last woman executed by the federal government was Ethel Rosenberg for giving the secrets
of the atomic bomb to the Soviet Union. Because her alleged

crimes occurred at the Northampton Veterans Administration Medical Center, a federal facility, Gilbert would be prosecuted under federal laws and therefore she was facing the death penalty. It was the same as if she committed a murder on an Army base.

The quiet college town of Northampton was abuzz with the scandalous case. Jurors who would have the power of life or death over Gilbert were selected from the local community. Out of a pool of eighty potential jurors, twelve jurors and six alternates had to be selected. Jury selection took four and a half weeks.

Our investigation amassed an enormous amount of paperwork. It included: thousands of pages of medical charts and nurses' notes, all gone over word by word by Bruce's Angels; Baden's autopsy notes and recordings made during the process; Rieders' toxicology report; Plante's investigative reports; Murphy's reports to his supervisors at the Massachusetts State Police; the notes compiled by the three nurses who first came forward with allegations against Gilbert; and more.

I was not able to be there for the entire trial. I still had an office to run back in New York and we had many other cases in the pipeline that had to be addressed. Those ID thieves, embezzlers, drug dealers, and fraudsters were not taking vacations because Kristen Gilbert was facing the death penalty for killing four patients. But I did not want to miss Welch's opening remarks. From the first day I met him, he demonstrated commitment and determination to find justice for the veterans who suffered at the hand of Gilbert. Now his time had come.

Opening remarks at trials are fascinating. It provides the jurors with a road map to where the prosecution and the defense hope to wind up at the end of the trial. Both sides lay out how they will prove their case, what witnesses will be called, and how easy it will be for the jury to rule in its favor. A prosecutor's opening remarks are like the first paragraph in a suspense novel: strong enough so you want to hear what comes next. The defense, on the other hand, wants you to reject this story as nothing more than nonsense.

The jurors and spectators analyze the cast of players as well. Jurors ask themselves if they like the attorneys. They wonder if the family and friends of the defendants are genuinely concerned and compassionate. Are the government agents honest and likable? The spectators are watching the jurors to see who's interested, who's taking notes, who's falling asleep, who's frowning, and who seems angry at the defendant or the government.

The Gilbert trial had all the elements of sensational court cases: a beautiful alleged murderess, a ditched husband, a handsome and confused boyfriend, betrayal by colleagues, damning testimony by experts, great detective work, and suspicious deaths. The courtroom was packed with media, friends and family, lawyers and their assistants, and several of those courthouse characters who hang around for months waiting for a big trial to occur. In Northampton, they had to wait around for years.

Gilbert's parents were in the gallery the first day and the following few days. I remember interviewing her father about his daughter's apparent problems at the hospital; he was more concerned that she was not disciplining her own children very well. Eventually, her parents stopped attending the sessions. I believe it was too difficult for them to watch the evidence pile up against their daughter. How can parents bear to see a child heading for death row?

The prosecution team was confident from day one. We had a strong case. We could prove the exhumed bodies contained epinephrine. We could follow the flow of drugs from the hospital pharmacy to where Gilbert had access to them. We could convincingly argue that she used the drug to create code situations so she could show off her nursing skills to the man she was obsessively consumed with—James Perrault. We did all of that.

She had a good defense at taxpayer's expense of more than one million dollars. Three court-appointed lawyers and medical experts and investigators would testify that our case was built on junk science. They also claimed it was an attempt to cover up hospital incompetence by throwing this highly competent, well-liked nurse to the dogs. What we did not have, they would drive home to the jury, was a witness. There was no one who could honestly testify they saw Gilbert steal epinephrine or give any of the victims a shot of the drug. Even the three nurses who complained about her to the VA administration to spark our investigation could not say they ever saw her do anything purposely that would have killed those four veterans.

But they could not debunk our star witness James Perrault, who testified that Gilbert told him during a phone call on July 10, 1996, that she had murdered patients. The defense argued that it was just the ranting of an emotionally upset woman desperate to say anything that would help save her quickly unraveling love affair with Perrault.

For the life of me, I could not understand how admitting to murder could make a person love you but that was all the defense they had regarding the confession. Veteran prosecutors observing the trial saw that confession as good as gold. "I never say any case is open and shut, but that admission to Perrault is all you guys really need," one veteran prosecutor told me after Perrault's dramatic appearance on the witness stand.

We hit one bump in the road when Rieders, at a pretrial hearing, conceded under oath that some of his mathematical calculations regarding the amounts of epinephrine found in the body were flawed. But no one argued that it wasn't epinephrine.

A friend of mine who teaches a class on criminal justice and was following the trial polled his students on the outcome. More than half voted for acquittal. Some of my colleagues in the VA OIG were betting on acquittal. I felt their attitude was more about the strong feelings they had that the IG community should not be involved in murder cases. These were some of the same managers who felt strongly that the IG community should only investigate fraud cases. That was water cooler conversation that followed me since the day I went to Northport VA Medical Center to interview Swango. After the Gilbert trial, that subject was a dead issue.

I heard it from my friends. The word was "Bruce Sackman thinks he's Sam Spade. He's pushing the envelope for his own ambition. What does he know about murder, he's in way over his head." It all got back to me. But I never saw my duty any other way. There was no homicide bureau in the VA. It was my job to enforce the laws of the organization and the civil and criminal laws that governed VA employees. It was not my job to call up the local police and ask them to investigate crime on VA property. I never thought I had a choice in the matter.

On March 14, 2001, after a six-month trial, the grim and tired-looking jury returned a verdict of guilty on three counts of first-degree murder, one count of second-degree murder, and two counts of assault. Gilbert was acquitted of the additional charges of assault with intent to kill a veteran and assault with intent to cause serious bodily injury in another veteran's death.

There was no celebration on our part. Hanging over the courtroom like a dark cloud was the fact that, upon conviction, the jury would now have to decide whether Gilbert would be executed for her crimes. To me, it was a dreadful process. She was guilty. I had no doubt about that.

All of a sudden at this time, people were asking me if I supported the death penalty. Friends, reporters, and even some on the prosecution team had differing opinions. It was conversation over coffee after the day in court. Days when I remained in New York, there was a constant buzz in the office about it. I had no easy answer. Personally, I was always opposed to the death penalty because it is too easy to make a mistake, as we see people exonerated after decades on death rows all over the country. But if someone had murdered my father in a VA hospital, I would want him or her executed. Years of pursuing Gilbert did not make the investigative team anxious for a death-penalty decision. The prosecutors made the argument for it with their characteristic style and determination and explained to the jury that the law implicitly called for death in this case. But we understood that the jury's decision would not be based on the law. It would be based on whether they accepted the death penalty as a punishment. My concern was more practical. I feared a decision in favor would bring on endless appeals that would tie up my resources for years.

After deliberating for a few days, the jury could not unanimously agree, so Gilbert's life would not be taken by the federal government.

Some months after the trial, one of the defense attorneys commented to the media that William Welch acted like a Nazi in his relentless pursuit of the death penalty. Nothing could be further from the truth. Welch performed his role as a government prosecutor and was as relieved as the rest of us when a final decision was handed down. I never heard him speak in private either in favor of, or against the death penalty for Gilbert.

On March 26, 2001, Gilbert was sentenced by Judge Michael Posner to four consecutive life terms for the murders of our nation's heroes at the Northampton VA Medical Center. In addition, she was sentenced to two twenty-year consecutive terms for assault with intent to kill two other veterans. Lastly, she was sentenced to one twenty-year count and one ten-year count to run concurrent with the life sentences for assaulting two other veteran patients. Gilbert was now in my rearview mirror. I was on my way to other things.

On June 27, 2003, while sitting at the conference table in my office, one of my special agents dropped a news story on my lap that almost knocked me to the floor. The headline in the Page Six section of the *New York Post* read, "Jailed Squeaky's Lesbian Lust." The article called it caged heat and reported "Lynette 'Squeaky' Fromme, who was sent to prison thirty years before for attempting to kill President Gerald Ford, has entered into a lesbian relationship in prison with convicted serial killer Kristen Gilbert." The article stated that they had so much in common that their close friendship blossomed into a love relationship.

Years after the trial, Judge Posner clearly used his experience presiding over the Gilbert death penalty case when he wrote a courtroom thriller drawn from real life. *The Hanging Judge* (Open Road, 2013) describes the fictitious case of a black drug dealer on trial in federal court for killing two people, told from the perspective of a judge rather than lawyers or police. Maybe truth is stranger than fiction!

To me, Kristen Gilbert was still seeking attention no matter what she had to do to get it. As of this writing, she is a forty-nine-year-old inmate at the minimum security Carswell Federal Medical Center in Fort Worth, Texas.

CHAPTER 14

Bruce's Angels

"Forensic nurses play an integral role in bridging the gap between law and medicine. They should be in each and every emergency room."

—JOSEPH BIDEN, former Vice President of the United States

My work on Swango and Gilbert brought me into contact for the first time with the great people who specialized in the field of forensic nursing. It was Doctor Baden who initially told me that I would need to bring at least two on board to help in the Swango investigation. Boy, was he correct! When I moved on to Gilbert, there was no doubt I would need them.

Forensic nurses are educated in and devote their skill to victims of violence and abuse. They are trained to care for the trauma that has been inflicted by sexual assailants, those who neglect, and those who inflict other forms of intentional injury. They are expert at collecting evidence, testimony, and other signs that a crime may have been committed. They are invaluable assets to law enforcement, from the cop on the

beat to prosecutors preparing cases against the vilest of perpetrators. Their education and experience make them excellent
witnesses at trials.

As *Forensic Nursing: A Handbook for Practice*" states,
"After attending to a patient's immediate needs, a forensic
nurse often collects evidence, provides medical testimony in
court, and consults with legal authorities."

Of course, in the cases on which I needed them to work,
there was not much they could do for the victims except see
that the person who harmed them was brought to justice. I
considered that a pretty big thing. I relied greatly on the information they gleaned from the medical records of the deceased,
which included the notes of all the attending doctors and especially those gems of knowledge known as "nurse's notes." I
was so effusive in my praise of their work that my regular team
of agents began calling them "Bruce's Angels." I took that as a
compliment to them.

Over the years, I have developed the greatest respect for
the nursing profession. Nurses of all disciplines are among the
most conscientious and dedicated persons I have ever met.
I've watched them with children, the elderly, injured, and everyone in between. It may sound corny, but they inspire me.
They are on the frontlines of our healthcare system. In the
Gilbert case, it was three heroic nurses who blew the whistle
on the killer loose in their hospital.

Nurses have not only been responsible for reporting suspicious events at healthcare institutions, they have also been
in the forefront of the investigation as well. Cops and prosecutors need a competent guide and interpreter to assist them
in their journey through the maze of hospital protocol. Most
criminal investigators have little or no medical background.
Most have no idea how a medical center operates, what data

is recorded in a patient's chart, how a pharmacy dispenses drugs, how a hospital peer review process works, or what is a DNR (Do Not Resuscitate) order. The investigator faces a considerable learning curve when first confronted with a suspicious death. In the early stages of the investigation, police depend on physicians and others to explain these processes. Unfortunately, police can become confused when inundated with too much information regarding a world with which they are unfamiliar. Here's where nurses come to the rescue.

I really knew very little about the workings of the medical side of a hospital before I began looking into the Swango case. Up until then, my concerns were more about what went on in the auditor's office or among the staff who handled cash and, of course, the complaints of ID theft, which did not necessarily bring me in touch with a doctor or nurse.

So I needed as much help at learning about what the doctors and nurses did as I did about Doctor Baden's expertise. The challenge for a forensic nurse is that he or she must explain complicated rules and medical observations to lay people. It requires thorough knowledge of medicine and the law to determine if something criminal occurred in the death of a patient.

It all begins with an understanding of hospital regulations and quality-of-care issues and evolves into the art of explaining medical procedures and medical terminology to nonmedical people. Nurses often reflect upon patient care from a different perspective than physicians or technicians, noting improprieties and spotting errors that other medical professionals miss. Nurses are knowledgeable about drug interactions and the appropriateness of prescriptions. All these skills are essential to the investigative team.

One brilliant forensic nurse, Mary Sullivan, developed a unique course for nurses entitled "Crime Scene Preservation and Death Investigation." In her course description Sullivan writes:

"After the first years of professional nursing practice, most nurses have mastered the skill of assessing the situation with one good look, i.e., monitors, IV, visitors, food tray, catheters, etc., and have prioritized the most important tasks that must be done immediately and usually without assistance. Any nurse with any direct patient care experience at all, has mastered the skill of doing two or three tasks at once without compromising any of them. Most nurses have this gold mine of information stored in their heads about signs and symptoms of hundreds of things that can go wrong with the human body as well as some amazing reflexes as to how to react in many types of emergencies. This gold mine of stored information and skills taken for granted are what makes nurses perfect candidates for crime scene teams and evidence management."

Sullivan continues,

"Let's get back to the "thinking skills" of a nurse. You walk into a patient's room and while your senses take in many bits of information, your brain pulls it all together. If it happens to be a crisis situation, your brain is already making assessments of what is wrong and what plan of action is required. You then methodically do what you are trained to do to handle the situation. And finally, you complete the documentation of the whole experience. All nurses get the message at one time or another that if it is not charted, it was not done. Further documentation must be objective and factual. Many nurses understand the "CYA" (cover your assets) concept when it comes to documentation: a careful summary of all facts, precise description, who was called, etc. Just in case the folks in the quality management department happen to pick your patient to review or that heaven forbid, a lawyer finds a reason to read the chart!"

A perfect example of the value of Bruce's Angels was a crucial development in the Gilbert case. One of our forensic nurses going through the files of a Gilbert victim noticed that there was no printout of an EKG that should have been given while working on the patient who had coded.

Gilbert had called in the code and was first to administer to the patient. She should have gotten at least one EKG reading as soon as possible. After all, she believed the patient was having a heart attack and that was the cause of death listed on the death certificate. Of course, Gilbert did not need an EKG since she knew the veteran was dying as a result of the shot of epinephrine she gave him. Those missing EKG printouts were crucial to the prosecution.

So, as I was ingesting all of this under the pressure of managing homicide investigations—plus what I was learning from Doctor Baden and detectives like Tom, Plante, and Murphy; and even from a major league prosecutor like Bill Welch—I wondered why none of these procedural elements were written down between the covers of a book or at least a manual.

I was beginning to understand this was a worldwide problem. Look what Swango got away with in Africa. Healthcare professionals were literally getting away with murder and no one was schooled on how to identify them not only after they killed but also, to catch them before they killed.

Of course, my new career direction was a favorite topic among my colleagues, and family and friends. It was fascinating in the way a highway crash is fascinating. People wanted details. It was more than morbid curiosity—my colleagues wanted to know how to stop the killing!

I understood that, as I compiled files filled with anecdotes and statistics, it was my obligation to share my knowledge. It was gruesome information, such as how much epinephrine it takes to kill a man, how succinylcholine is stolen from a hospital pharmacy, and how a code emergency is created. I just didn't want to tell war stories. I wanted to produce a road map on how to successfully investigate these cases.

What troubled me, and still does to this day, is that these perpetrators are not identified until they have killed numerous patients, and someone finally notices the dramatic increase in the death rate of a particular ward or unit. The killer nurse, Donald Harvey, said that after he killed his first sixteen patients, and no one noticed, he felt he was ordained by God to continue killing. Why did it take sixteen victims before the staff noticed something wrong? Why, in my long VA career up to this point, were there only three identified instances of MSKs?

These thoughts did not depress me. I did not lose sleep worrying that an MSK might be at work at that moment in a rural VA hospital somewhere in America. In fact, I was energized by the course my career was now on. And I was excited by the feeling that was traveling through the entire IG community, that an organization like the VA OIG could successfully investigate the most bizarre and complicated homicide cases that were so far out of the usual realm of fraud, waste, and abuse with which we commonly dealt. I was very proud of my work and the work of my colleagues. When the VA OIG Special Agent in Charge of the Midwest region called to ask me some advice about a case of a suspected MSK named Richard Williams, I was certain I was fulfilling a much-needed service for America's veterans and raising the profile of my own profession.

That phone call convinced me I needed to create a concise, evidence-based road map leading to early awareness of an MSK at work, from investigating the killer, to prosecuting the killer. I decided to call it The Red Flags Protocol (RFP). As of April 2018, my RFP presentation is in demand at health-care-related events all over the world.

CHAPTER 15

The Red Flags Protocol

"The impossible could not have happened,
therefore the impossible must be possible in spite of
appearances."

—AGATHA CHRISTIE, *Murder on the Orient Express*

The work of the forensic nurses is indispensable in the investigation of a crime. But unless we take seriously the clues they discover, we are wasting our time and energy and giving a green light to murderous healthcare workers who know how to hide the evidence of their crimes.

All nurses are the Army Rangers of healthcare workers whose mission is to heal our wounds and deliver us back in good health to our loved ones. They lead the way. They are in front of the front lines. They hear all and see all that goes on around them and there are none better positioned to report trouble brewing. Those nurses in mind led me to develop what I earlier alluded to as the Red Flags Protocol (RFP). It should be part of the curriculum in every nursing school and medical school.

I am first and foremost an investigator, a homicide detective who arrives when the ICU has been turned into a crime scene. I am charged with finding the killer responsible for the death of a patient. But no detective studies a crime without having the thought about how it could have been prevented. Crime prevention is the major function of a police department. All cops wished they had less work to do; it means there is less crime. The RFP shows both sides of the coin. A clue can lead to solving the mystery of a "who done it" and it can provide a course of action that may prevent the crime in the first place.

I unveiled the RFP at a conference sponsored by the New York State Police following the highly-publicized Gilbert trial. I received a standing ovation, led by the forensic nurses in the audience.

I began with a shocking statement, "Hospitals are the perfect hunting grounds for those bent on serial killing."

Consider the scene of the crime. The victims have not been found dead in an alley in a seedy neighborhood on the other side of the tracks. There are no flashing police lights or the sounds of sirens rushing to the rescue. That is what we expect from a typical murder scene. But the scenes I investigated took place in hospitals. The victims were surrounded by medical professionals fighting to save their lives. Or they were found dead. Yet, just as the body in the alley might have been surrounded by clues, so were the victims in my cases, and those clues could also lead to the possibility of preventing that death, stopping the killer before the act.

Nothing makes hospital administrators cringe more than the thought of a staff member intentionally harming a patient. Administrators will argue that errors occur, and patients are unexpectedly harmed through malpractice or unexpected complications. To treat an ICU like a crime scene simply because of a suspicious medical event will send the wrong message to visitors, patients, and staff. Staff may feel that they are now subject to criminal prosecution for an honest mistake. Furthermore, the establishment of something akin to a crime scene criminal investigation, many believe, will only provide useful information for a strong defense in the inevitable lawsuits that are to follow.

Because of the career I chose and the job I held, my investigations concerned suspicious deaths in Veterans Administration Medical Centers. At first, I worried the VA seemed to be afflicted with this peculiar circumstance. But I quickly learned that it is a problem that afflicts every type of hospital, private or public.

Hospital managers have a well-documented history of defending employees suspected of intentionally harming patients. They are afraid that bad publicity and potential lawsuits will follow formal investigations, especially if conducted by outside authorities like a district attorney. When the police or DA get involved, a record of their activity is a public record. The media will find out about it and sensational stories will result. They are right to fear that but sweeping the problem under the rug is not a solution.

If only an in-house investigation is conducted, it is likely that none of the investigative team members will have any forensic experience. Therefore, the likely conclusion of such an investigation will be that the patient died of one or more of his or her documented medical conditions and, therefore, the death could be attributed to a natural disease process.

Silence and the failure to communicate to even other hospital administrations is like pouring salt in the wounds. It makes enablers out of people who should be stopping suspect healthcare workers in their tracks. The same holds true for law enforcement agencies that do not share information that might lead to tracking suspected killers.

Journalist Thomas Hargrove studied how many victims or serial killers might go unnoticed, allowing the killer to get away with murder. A 2017 article in the *Atlantic* reported on his findings.

Believing he could create an algorithm that would enable an investigator to identify serial killings, Hargrove dove into the FBI's annual homicide reports, according to the article. His "Murder Accountability Project" eventually assembled a database indicating there are an outstanding two hundred and twenty thousand unsolved murders in the U.S. each year. Hargrove attributed two thousand to the work of serial killers. But Hargrove's algorithm, according to the article, concluded that there are actually twenty-seven thousand more homicides then the FBI's records disclosed. Hargrove attributes the difference in numbers to "linkage blindness." Law enforcement is not talking to one other.

"The only way a murder is linked to a common offender is if the two investigators get together at a water cooler and talk about their cases and discover commonalities," said Hargrove. I asked Hargrove if his algorithm can detect MSKs. He told me that "the threat posed by medical serial killers is that their victims often are not detected as homicides—at least, not immediately. They are active within hospitals or other medical facilities where death is common."

Hargrove said that the government, using Medicare and Medicaid records, has tried to identify facilities that have an unusually high fatality rate. Hospitals say this effort is inherently unfair. "Our methods employ an algorithm that can detect clusters of homicides of similar type within a similar geography that have exceptionally low clearance rates," Hargrove said. "To my knowledge, our methods have never issued a warning over a medical series (killers). My suspicion is that's because the killings were not originally reported as homicides at the time the death occurred. So-called "Angel of Mercy" deaths and other types of medical serial killers represent a truly horrifying threat to public safety since their victims are invisible to law enforcement."

This may seem cynical but from my experience it is on the mark. His algorithm can identify clusters of unsolved murders, which are related by the method, location, time of the murder, and the victim's gender. It's sort of like the Red Flags in my protocol.

The article reports Hargrove utilized his software to discover and alert the police department in Gary, Indiana, of fifteen unsolved strangulations in the area. "It was absolute radio silence," he said. "They would not talk about the possibility that there was an active serial killer."

When people die in a hospital unexpectedly, hospital administration must not be afraid to consider there is a link to the deaths and that link might be one of their own employees. They must share their concerns regardless of the consequences.

When I started the Swango investigation, there were more than forty sudden-death injectable poisons available on a VA ward. Many of these drugs are of a type considered "non-detectable" or are generally not looked for during an autopsy. In most of these cases, no autopsy is even ever performed. Since the patients had medical problems that eventually could have resulted in death, absent of any evidence of wrongdoing, it was customary to accept one of those ailments as the official cause of death. Even if an autopsy were performed, it would not have revealed any of the forty instant-death chemicals because there was no reason to suspect their use. With IV lines, feeding tubes, and syringes being utilized all the time, poisons could be administered with relative ease and non-detection.

The solution is in the Red Flags Protocol and what it can teach us about prevention. Ignoring those suspicions is precisely what MSKs depend on. They expect that instead of calling in law enforcement, at worst, hospital management might give them a bad report, but then help them find a new job somewhere else. That is what happened in the Michael Swango and Douglas Harvey cases.

Here is what I determined was the best way to identify MSKs:

The A-To-Z of My Red Flags Protocol

A. The rate of death increases when treated by the suspect. (Swango, Gilbert)

B. The suspect worked the "graveyard" shift, was alone with the patient, and screened off by the "Murder Curtain" at time of death. (Swango, Gilbert)

C. The suspect is uncannily accurate in predicting a patient's death. (This is extremely important to note because it is mostly anecdotal and most victims are on their way to recovery.

D. The patient's death was unexpected, and the family was not present at his/her bedside. (Swango, Gilbert)

E. The death certificate cites the patient's last known illness or a catchall like cardiac arrest. (Swango, Gilbert)

F. Fellow employees report allegations, not management. (Swango, Gilbert)

G. Suspect often continues patient care during the investigation, removed only after allegations become public. (Swango fled to Africa, Gilbert resigned from the hospital)

H. There is rarely an eyewitness to the crime. (One circumstantially in Swango, none in Gilbert)

I. The weapon of choice is usually a "sudden-death" chemical readily available on the ward, and often undetectable or not looked for at an autopsy. (Swango, Gilbert)

J. Suspect is usually charming and friendly but has difficulty in personal relationships. (Swango, Gilbert)

K. Suspect displays questionable dress code or mannerisms. (Gilbert)

L. Suspect receives good written reviews from supervisors. (Swango, Gilbert)

M. Suspect collects books and videos regarding horrible deaths. (Swango)

N. Suspect never expresses remorse at the death of a patient. (Swango, Gilbert)

O. Suspect is considered an excellent performer in an emergency, especially during code incidents. (Swango, Gilbert)

P. Suspect is involved in an inordinate amount of code incidents. (Swango, Gilbert)

Q. Suspect craves fame. (Gilbert)

R. There is evidence the suspect killed, or attempted to kill, when he or she was off duty. (Swango, Gilbert)

S. Initial review usually finds insufficient evidence to assess the case. Management buys in quickly to avoid damage to reputation. (Swango, Gilbert)

T. Syringes, IV lines, and feeding tubes are most likely entry points for the poison. (Swango, Gilbert)

U. If a code is called, EKG printouts should be in the file. (Gilbert)

V. Witnesses report seeing suspect with patient before death. (Swango)

W. Suspect was given pejorative nickname by colleagues. (Swango, Gilbert)

X. Prior employment records show questionable incidents and recommendations. (Swango, Gilbert)

Y. Even in the face of evidence to the contrary, suspect insists the patient died of natural causes. (Gilbert)

Z. Killing is nonconfrontational. (Swango, Gilbert)

It does not take a neurosurgeon to figure out that close and ongoing monitoring of behavior by all staff—doctors, nurses, and all kinds of assistants who have access to drugs and patients—can prevent MSKs from achieving their desire to kill. Most importantly, hospital brass must listen to their staff when allegations are made. Michael Swango, Kristen Gilbert, Donald Harvey, and others were left free to kill even after hospital brass was warned.

CHAPTER 16

The Hall of Shame

> "Things that are done, it is needless to speak about...
> things that are past, it is needless to blame."
>
> —CONFUCIUS, *The Analects of Confucius*

I agree with Confucius up to a point. A homicide investigator must find someone to blame for a murder. And when I look at the bigger picture of how MSKs got away with murder, I find the blame usually falls on hospital officials who refuse to look at the facts presented to them for fear of damage to their institutions. But rather than focusing on placing blame, I hope my work sheds light on how to stop MSKs. As I learned about MSKs who killed way before Swango or Gilbert came on the scene, I am confident genuine adherence to my RFP would have at least slowed them down, perhaps stopped them completely. I believe I could have saved countless lives.

One afternoon at a police seminar in Manhattan, I met a Scotland Yard detective who gave a short talk on the British MSK Doctor Harold Shipman. After the conference, I asked the detective to join me for a cup of coffee.

We talked as we walked along Tenth Avenue near John Jay College of Criminal Justice. He was quite animated. He told me that 459 patients died under Shipman's care between 1971 and 1998. Of these, Scotland Yard believed three hundred were murdered by the doctor. As we walked, the detective made his point by drawing attention to a building along the way. "It was as if he killed fifty in that building, then one hundred in that building, and fifty over there in that building."

He made his point very well. Imagine if instead of choosing hospitals for his hunting ground, Shipman prowled the streets of New York. He would have wiped out whole neighborhoods.

As a young man, Shipman was an outstanding athlete and very close to his mother. She died of lung cancer when he was seventeen. Shipman watched his mother suffer in extreme pain for many months. As she progressively lost her battle to survive, a doctor treated her regularly at her home with morphine injections, which eased her pain as she slipped away.

I have no doubt that his MO in killing patients was influenced by the experience of watching his mother's painful losing battle. Only the morphine eased her struggle. But, as I learned, he was no "Angel of Mercy." His weapon of choice, supported by evidence obtained through the process of exhumations and autopsies, was heroin, and it is commonly used in some countries to control pain. But Shipman was injecting lethal doses. A difference between him and, say, Swango or Harvey, was that he had his own office and he treated patients at their homes. It would have been difficult to monitor his morphine supply, which might have raised a red flag.

However, it was another red flag that eventually led to his demise.

In March 1998, a nurse and a funeral home owner expressed concern to the coroner in the South Manchester area of London that there was an unusually high death rate among Shipman's patients. They noticed that the possible victims were mostly elderly women and that Shipman had been requesting an unusual number of cremation forms. I guess he figured, no body, no exhumation down the road.

The police investigated for about one month but could deduce no evidence that merited criminal charges. There were no forensic nurses or pathologists involved in the investigation. Shipman continued seeing patients during the investigation, something that the RFP warns against. My Scotland Yard friend believed Shipman killed several more people while the investigation continued.

In June 1998, a woman named Kathleen Grundy, seventy-eight, was found dead in her home shortly after a visit from Shipman. He was the last person to see her alive and signed the death certificate listing "old age" as the cause of death. Again, the RFP says the killer is usually the last person to see the victim before death and attributes the demise to a natural cause.

But Grundy would be the last of the monster's victims. Her daughter, a lawyer, learned that her mother left a will that excluded her and her children but instead left a small fortune to Shipman.

The daughter went to the police, who this time took a closer look at Shipman. Working with a forensics team, they exhumed Grundy's body and searched for traces of a drug that if used would be difficult to find. They found traces of morphine. A search of his home did not turn up books on poisons or *Tales from the Crypt* horror stories. But eventually, a typewriter that they linked to a false will was discovered.

For two years, investigators looked at all the deaths certified by Shipman during his career. The prosecution settled on 250 patients who died at the hands of this doctor. Eighty percent of them were elderly women. He was arrested on September 7, 1998.

The prosecution's case was that Shipman enjoyed exercising a power of life or death over his victims. He could care less about being an "Angel of Mercy," putting them out of their misery. And he robbed them as well, perhaps to feed his own drug addiction. After he administered the deadly shot, he stole their jewelry. Thousands of dollars in jewelry was discovered in his garage after he was arrested. And in at least the case that led to his arrest, he convinced an elderly widow to have a will drawn up separate from her family, so she could leave him money.

In January 2000, a jury found Shipman guilty of fifteen murders, just a small percentage of how many investigators believed he committed. He was sentenced to life plus four years for the forgery of the will. Shipman hanged himself in his prison cell in January 2004, one day shy of his fifty-eighth birthday.

If you are in London you might pay a visit to the memorial garden to Shipman's victims. Called the Garden of Tranquility, it is located in Hyde Park. Shipman is the only British physician known to have murdered patients. But I am certain there are others.

Following the Shipman conviction, the British health/legal system instituted some changes similar to the Red Flags Protocol. Shipman's macabre story has been well documented in the media, websites like Wikipedia, and court records. But hearing about it from that Scotland Yard detective made me even more proud of the work we accomplished on Swango and Gilbert and validated my work on the Red Flags Protocol.

America's equivalent to Shipman, in terms of numbers of victims, is Charles Cullen. He was a New Jersey nurse who confessed to killing forty patients during his sixteen-year career by drawing the "Murder Curtain" around their bedside and adding drugs to their IVs. Nobody really knows how many he killed but investigators I have spoken with over the years all agree his victims numbered in the hundreds. They also agree an institutionalized Red Flags Protocol could have saved many lives.

As more of his life was probed by psychiatrists, journalists, and detectives, it is pretty much accepted that he probably killed hundreds of people. He would not give an exact number because in his words he "lived in a fog." That admission would put him at the top of the list of MSKs.

Cullen told detectives he killed because he wanted the patients to be spared the frightful experience of being coded or going into cardiac arrest. But, don't believe it. He enjoyed killing people!

As reported in newspapers, websites, and books about Cullen, he experienced a childhood that could not have prepared him for anything but a life of bizarre misery.

He was raped by his father, who died while Cullen was still a child. At the age of nine, he tried suicide by drinking chemicals from a chemistry set. When he was seventeen, his mother died in a car crash while his sister was driving. Over the years, he told psychiatrists he fantasized about stealing drugs from a hospital where he worked and using them to kill himself. Once he took a pair of scissors and stabbed himself in the head. Ironically, he was saved by emergency surgery. He eventually tried to end his own life twenty times. Many of these attempts occurred while he was working as a nurse. They were red flags that were ignored by administrators. He was allowed to continue his nursing career.

He was a high school dropout but apparently found his place in the U.S. Navy Submarine Service, rising in the ranks to petty officer third class, and bore the responsibilities of a member of a Poseidon missile team. It's hard for me to imagine he passed the Navy psychological profiles that go with such important duties because he was clearly a troubled seaman.

One day, he showed up wearing a surgical gown, latex gloves, and mask he had stolen from a medical cabinet. He wore them through his entire shift on the missiles. That act got him transferred to a supply ship, where he soon tried to commit suicide. In 1984, after his seventh military suicide attempt, the Navy finally understood he was a bad risk and he was discharged.

Nevertheless, he was able to enroll in New Jersey's Mountainside School of Nursing. Three years later, he landed a nursing position at St. Barnabas Medical Center in Livingston, New Jersey, where he almost immediately began administering lethal doses of drugs to patients. That same year, he married Adrienne Taub, with whom he had two daughters.

He later admitted committing his first murder at St. Barnabas in 1988. A local judge had been admitted suffering from an allergic reaction to a prescribed blood thinner. Cullen gave him a lethal dose of insulin though his IV tube. Eventually, Cullen admitted to killing eleven patients at St. Barnabas, including an AIDS patient. Overdoses of insulin was his weapon of choice. No one took notice of an unusual death rate among his patients.

Finally, in 1992, an internal investigation into some contamination of IV bags was conducted, which began pointing at Cullen. There were no exhumations, no autopsies, no search for killer drugs. Cullen was simply asked to leave.

This erratic behavior did not prevent him from landing a job at Warren Hospital in Phillipsburg, New Jersey. By his own admission, he soon killed three elderly women with overdoses of the heart medication, digoxin. His final victim at Warren said that a "sneaky male nurse" had injected her as she slept, but family members and other healthcare workers dismissed her comments. The RFP warns against doing that.

In December 1993, Cullen left Warren Hospital, and movinged on to Hunterdon Medical Center in New Jersey, where he worked in the intensive care/cardiac unit for three years.

During the first two years, Cullen claims he did not murder anyone. When he was arrested in 2003, the hospital claimed records covering Cullen's work had been destroyed. There was nothing for forensic investigators to pore over. Are we supposed to believe that? Disgraceful! Eventually, Cullen admitted to murdering five patients during that period in 1996. Weapon of choice: overdoses of digoxin.

Over the next four years, thanks to a nationwide shortage of nurses, Cullen was able to find work in various places in Pennsylvania and New Jersey. In 1992, he showed up in the cardiac care unit at St. Luke's Hospital in Bethlehem, Pennsylvania. He later admitted he killed five patients and attempted to kill two others while working there.

He was getting away with murder at St. Luke's until a colleague discovered unused vials of drugs in a disposal can. The drugs had no use or value outside of the hospital. The administration investigated and Cullen was accused of trying to steal the drugs. He was fired in 2002, but even if they suspected he was stealing the drugs so he could use them to kill patients, the hospital did not call in the police to investigate.

Cullen's colleagues had had enough. Seven nurses complained to the Lehigh County District Attorney in Pennsylvania that they believed Cullen killed patients at St. Luke's. Their evidence was straight out of the RFP. They argued that Cullen worked 20 percent of the hours on their ward but was present for nearly 66 percent of the deaths. The DA spent nine months investigating but did not follow the RFP and did not have the expertise to develop an airtight case. He dropped the case. I wish he had called me for help.

Cullen found a job in September 2002 in the critical care unit at the Somerset Medical Center in Somerville, New Jersey. Over the next nine months, according to his own admissions, he murdered eight more patients and attempted to murder another one. While his drug of choice was digoxin, he occasionally added insulin to his deadly arsenal.

Soon things began to unravel for the monster. An astute administrator noticed the hospital's computer systems showed that Cullen was accessing the records of patients to whom he was not assigned. Coworkers were seeing him in patients' rooms. Computerized drug-dispensing cabinets were showing that Cullen was requesting medications that patients had not been prescribed. These are all red flags straight out of my protocol.

Then in July 2003, the executive director of the New Jersey Poison Information & Education System warned Somerset Medical Center officials that at least four of the suspicious overdoses reported in their hospital indicated the possibility that an employee was killing patients. But the hospital put off contacting authorities until October. By then, Cullen had killed another five patients and attempted to kill a sixth.

State officials penalized the hospital for failing to report a nonfatal insulin overdose in August. The overdose had been administered by Cullen. When Cullen's final victim died of low blood sugar in October, the medical center alerted state authorities. Surprise, surprise, an investigation into Cullen's employment history revealed past suspicions about his involvement with prior deaths. Why did it take almost a decade for someone to check his job history?

Somerset Medical Center fired Cullen on October 31, 2003, for lying on his job application, the same offense that led to Swango's downfall. The local police were now determined to bring him down and kept on him after he left the job.

Cullen was arrested on one count of murder and one count of attempted murder on December 14, 2003. That same day, he admitted to the murder of two other patients at Somerset.

In April 2004, Cullen pleaded guilty in a New Jersey court to killing thirteen patients and attempting to kill two others by lethal injection while employed at Somerset. As part of his plea agreement, he promised to cooperate with authorities if they did not seek the death penalty for his crimes. A month later, he pleaded guilty to the murder of three more patients in New Jersey.

In November 2004, Cullen pleaded guilty in a Pennsylvania court to killing six patients and trying to kill three others.

On March 2, 2006, Cullen was sentenced to eleven consecutive life sentences in New Jersey, to be ineligible for parole for 397 years. He is held at New Jersey State Prison in Trenton, New Jersey. When you add his convictions in Pennsylvania, Cullen is serving eighteen life sentences.

I read Cullen's history in the popular media and I have discussed the cases with countless investigators in and out of the VA. We're in total agreement that adherence to the RFP or some similar version of it would have stopped Cullen in his tracks not long after he murdered his first victim.

CHAPTER 17

Angel of Mercy...Not

"I did not become a nurse so I could be an Angel of Mercy."

—NURSE RICHARD WILLIAMS

I first heard of Richard Williams during a break at the Swango sentencing. Over coffee near the courthouse, my boss, VA Inspector General Richard Griffin, asked me if I had heard about a case in Missouri where a nurse at the Harry S. Truman Memorial Veterans' Hospital was charged with killing a number of patients. Apparently, the FBI and local prosecutors did not have enough evidence to bring him to trial even though they exhumed the bodies of thirteen veterans.

I did know about this case. It was the reason the FBI passed on the Gilbert case. I read something about it in a widely distributed report from Griffin's office, but I was knee-deep in the Swango case at the time and did not pay as much attention to it as I would have liked. Now in the summer of 2001, I had put both Swango and Gilbert in prison and my interest and expertise in MSKs was being noticed by my colleagues throughout the VA and by law enforcement around the world.

At a one-day conference in Manhattan, I talked to an FBI agent who expressed his frustration over working on the Williams' case in never getting the nurse indicted. He told me the family of one of the alleged victims filed a wrongful death suit against the government; in 1998 there was a civil trial, which was ruled in favor of the family. But, he said, "That killer nurse is still working."

"You should take a look at this," he said. I left the conference determined to review any files the VA OIG had on this nurse named Richard Williams. But the greatest terrorist attack on America's soil stopped us in our tracks. On September 11, 2001, terrorists brought down the World Trade Center towers not far from my Manhattan office.

Like everyone else, where I was and what I was doing is forever embedded in my mind. I was sitting at my desk at 201 Varick Street—about twenty blocks north of the World Trade Center complex—on the telephone with an executive in my Boston office; one of my agents stuck his head in my door, saying, "Boss, a plane just hit the World Trade Center." I told the agent in Boston I would get back to her and with a few staffers in tow, went down to the street to look at the unfolding horror.

From the street in front of our office building, tremendous damage to Tower One was clearly visible. Not a small plan, I thought and *no accident on a crystal clear day like today.* I froze in place when we saw the second plane hit. I could not process what I was seeing. Within minutes, we gasped as people jumped off the towering roof to save themselves from the flames. It is an image I'll never forget.

Someone on the corner pointed to the building and screamed, "The Jews are to blame for this." That comment did not sit well with me, but this was not time for political debate. I ran upstairs and gathered everyone who was available and dispatched them to the nearest VA medical center, at Twenty-Third Street and First Avenue in Manhattan, with the orders to give any help they could to the hospital staff dealing with victims. I did not have to say it twice. The office emptied in about a minute. I informed DC what we were doing and then followed my people out the door.

We waited at the hospital all day. But our help was not needed. Practically no one showed up. The horror of the day was compounded when we realized there were not going to be many injured survivors. Those that were trapped above the collision points died. Those below who escaped were not injured badly. We understood they were cared for on the scene or taken to closer public hospitals. We went home that night not really sure what our role would be in the following days. We were federal law enforcement officers. We carried weapons and knew how to use them. We were anxious to do whatever was necessary to either save lives or go after the terrorists who perpetrated this crime.

The following day, I was able to get close to the impact zone. It was dangerous to get around without boots and a mask. The worst part to me was seeing the firemen in a daze over what had happened. They lost more than three hundred comrades. I wanted to go over to offer my condolences, but it was difficult to find the right words.

I could see this was no place for white-collar crime investigators. It was extraordinarily dangerous and very easy for the untrained to get hurt. After a few hours, I ordered my team out of there. Some agents were angry with me, but I thought we might actually cause more harm than good being so ill-equipped and ill-prepared for the job ahead. I knew there would be better roles for us to play in the days ahead.

Years later, it was determined that if you spent a considerable amount of time at ground zero on the first three days you had the highest possibility of developing some "9/11-related illness." After getting a ration of shit from some agents, eventually they all realized that I may have saved their lives by that decision.

That weekend, Eileen and I went in to the city to the National Guard armory to help the families of victims find a way to cope with their tragedy. It was very emotional work.

Soon, the debris from the site was transported by barge and truck to the Staten Island landfill. I volunteered my team to go through the debris, but this time suited up and properly equipped. We all took turns down at the site for months on end, almost an entire year. We were assigned to search the debris from Building Seven, which had housed federal offices. We were looking for personal items like wallets or watches—things that might help identify victims. It was important work. We were doing what we could to help bring closure to the families of the victims. I thought it was akin to what I did with the MSKs. The families of the killers found a measure of peace when Swango and Gilbert were sent to prison for life.

The landfill had been an Environmental Protection Agency (EPA) disaster before they dumped everything up there. I remember the sanitation workers at the bottom of the hill stating, "You guys are going up there? We don't even go up there!" The area was otherworldly. It was filled with fire trucks, other vehicles, and building parts smashed like pancakes that were unrecognizable.

One day I took Doctor Baden and my boss, Richard Griffin, up to the site. I remember Griffin saying, "Bruce, this would have never happened if the FBI had done its job." He was angry and shared my dislike for the Bureau, but on that score, it's debatable and that was not the right time or place for that argument.

I worked on and off at the landfill for about eighteen months. When I returned home, I felt a pressure in my chest. It would subside after a few days. When we first arrived, there was nothing at the landfill site except for an Army National Guard Mobile Army Surgical Hospital (MASH) tent. Tom Valery arranged for a medical trailer to be brought from the Northport VA to help provide specialized support. Of all of us, Tom probably spent the most time at the site, being a volunteer firefighter himself. At the end of our assignment, all our government vehicles had to be destroyed because the soot and ash from the site seemed to magically stick to their bottom and could not be removed. It got so bad that we had to ride with the windows open because the smell became un-bearable. And this stuff was in our lungs!

Now, once a year I get examined at the 9/11 clinic, which was established to treat first responders. So far so good.

During the eighteen months I was absorbed with the World Trade Center, I never lost my interest in Richard Williams. I read all the available reports on the investigation that went nowhere. I also read a report by Griffin's office that stated the victims could have been given a paralyzing drug. I spoke to some people at Truman in Missouri who echoed the same sentiment but said there was no physical evidence to back up the instinct. I knew they did not have Doctor Rieders' machine when the investigation was underway in the mid-1990s.

The more I read, the more confident I grew that I could make a difference in this case. I was bursting with knowledge and enthusiasm. I called Griffin and just about said, "Put me in, Coach!" He understood and respected my zeal but was not anxious to get mired in the case at that time. After all, the FBI investigated it and local prosecutors tried hard to make a criminal case but had failed. There was already a civil trial ruled in favor of the family. Griffin didn't see much reason to get involved at this point.

But I argued with him that with Baden, Rieders, and Bruce's Angels aboard, we could find new evidence and get an indictment and a criminal trial. He reminded me that Baden and Rieders were being used by the FBI and could not turn up the goods needed. I enjoyed this back and forth with Griffin. He was a very intelligent and decent guy. He wanted the best for the VA.

Eventually I sold this project to my bosses as nothing more than taking a second look at the patients' folders. I did not see how that could hurt. If we uncovered something, we could then collectively discuss the next move. Griffin agreed with the informal approach and gave me the green light. Shortly thereafter, the medical records arrived at my office in New York City.

In November of 2001, I received tissue samples of ten of the thirteen veterans whose bodies had been exhumed in 1993 when the FBI was running its investigation. The samples were turned over by the Bureau to the Boone County Medical Examiner in Missouri in 1998 and were kept there until I requested them. I was greatly encouraged by the Boone County ME's timely response to my request. So far, not a person I spoke to who had a part in the investigation of Williams did not think he was a killer. By now, I knew Richard Williams backwards and forwards and was ready to prove what everyone thought to be true.

CHAPTER 18

Deaf Ears

"Always do right. This will gratify some people
and astonish the rest."

—MARK TWAIN

Richard Williams was a nurse at the Truman Veterans'
Memorial Hospital in Columbia, Missouri. He was
charged with killing ten of his patients but never convicted. I
tried my best to put him behind bars for life.

This is what I knew: In 1992, there was an alarming increase in the murder rate in the twenty-seven-bed Ward C of
the Truman Veterans' Hospital. The patients were dying on the
midnight shift, which was typically served by just one nurse.
The victims were not patients expected to die according to their
families or the medical staff. These unexpected deaths were noticed by other nurses in the hospital, who voiced their concerns
to the administration. Their voices fell on deaf ears. One of
the complaining nurses even asked for reassignment to another
ward but was refused.

The one nurse assigned to Ward C was a newly-licensed registered nurse, Richard Williams. He was often in charge of the ward from midnight to eight o'clock in the morning. In a one-month period since Williams arrived at the ward, there were a dozen unexpected deaths. Usually, Ward C might average three in a month.

Incredibly, I learned Williams had been fired from his previous job at St. John's Hospital in Springfield, Missouri, after it was discovered he allegedly withheld medicine from patients and falsified charts to indicate they had received their proper dosages. However, human resources officials at that hospital were tight-lipped about Williams' firing, and while I believe some of the top people at Truman knew of his past record, they hired him anyway.

By summer of that year, the hospital's quality improvement staff could no longer ignore the rising death rate. They took their concerns to J.L. Kurzejeski, the hospital director, and Doctor Gordon Christensen, the associate chief of staff for research.

Christensen took the complaints seriously and did a comprehensive job of investigating them. He began by charting the time and date of fifty-five deaths and noted who the nurse on duty was at the time. Historically, hospital statistics show that most patient deaths occur around eight o'clock in the morning, with the numbers peaking in the afternoon. Patients seldom die in hospitals between midnight and three o'clock in the morning. Christensen's research determined that out of fifty-five patients who died on the ward between March 8 and August 22, 1992, forty-five were under Williams' care. Patients were an outrageously twenty times more likely to die if nurse Williams was caring for them compared to any other nurses in the hospital. Without any other way to explain the increase in the death rate, Christensen concluded the patients in question were being murdered. Putting two and two together, my conclusion after reading Christensen's report was that Richard Williams was an MSK.

Most doctors at Truman never noticed Williams before the rumors he was killing patients began to spread. He was described to investigators as balding, soft-spoken and having a soft, fat face and a slight lisp. Williams usually kept to himself. "There was nothing special about him, nothing that stood out," one nurse remembered. One doctor described him as "creepy looking and dumpy with big shark eyes."

Then a series of events happened that I knew by now were typical reactions inside VA hospitals to the stunning news that a healthcare professional was an evil force at work in their wards.

Armed with Christensen's research, Director Kurzejeski called an emergency meeting of the hospital's highest-ranking staffers in which he laid out the gruesome conclusion of the report. Following Kurzejeski's presentation, he was asked by his colleagues to call the police. He flat-out rejected that recommendation.

I gleaned from the VA OIG's file that Doctor Edward Adelstein, a hospital pathologist and deputy medical examiner of Boone County, said he was present during a telephone conversation between Kurzejeski and the VA regional chief of staff regarding the matter. Adelstein said the chief of staff specifically warned Kurzejeski that the last time a VA medical center called in the FBI, the director and the chief of staff were fired. He then asked Kurzejeski if that was something he wanted his bosses to do—call in the FBI. Kurzejeski responded, "No." He clearly got the message that the regional chief of staff was delivering. *Button it up! Keep it within the hospital!* Officially, Williams was cleared of any wrongdoing.

As I read through the file I could not understand Kurzejeski's next move. I understood he was not going to call law enforcement, but he might have at least found something for Williams to do that did not bring him in contact with patients. Instead, he assigned another nurse to work alongside Williams. I concede that when this second nurse was on duty, the death rate declined. But any day a second nurse was unavailable to work with Williams, the death rate increased dramatically. I just found this unbelievable incompetence at work.

Within a month of Christensen's report and the cover-up, the local news media learned of the suspicious deaths at Truman and forced Kurzejeski to come forward to answer questions about them. On September 30, 1992, he held a news conference to report that an internal investigation found "the patients' deaths are attributed to one or more of the patients' underlying medical problems." In effect, Williams was cleared but at least now he was assigned to clerical work.

Kurzejeski even wrote a letter to Williams telling him that a board of inquiry found no evidence of wrongdoing on his part. This flew in the face of Christensen's analysis. But the cover-up continued. It was embarrassing for me to read the report. I loved the VA. It was my passion to work for them. I knew how much good our medical centers had done for our heroes over the years. I knew that the overwhelming number of employees, from receptionists to surgeons, were selfless, highly-skilled individuals. To this day, I can't wrap my mind around hospital bosses at the highest levels thinking a cover-up of a murder, or in Williams' case, possibly numerous murders, served anyone's purpose except the killer's. It made me sick.

Then on October 5, 1992, two heroic nurses secretly contacted the FBI. After a meeting, the Bureau did the right thing and brought the local VA OIG aboard. They seized all pertinent records from the hospital and contacted Doctor Baden to conduct forensic autopsies. The aggressive move sent shockwaves through the VA system. From February to March of 1993, the bodies of thirteen veterans were exhumed and the FBI laboratory tested tissue samples. Baden concluded that ten of these veterans did not die from natural disease processes, as Kurzejeski told reporters at that news conference and as listed on their death certificates. But the actual cause of death could not be determined.

The FBI and VA OIG interviewed everyone connected in any way to the investigation, but examination of tissue samples from the exhumed bodies was seriously delayed by the Bureau's need to respond to two major events—first, the 1993 bombing of the World Trade Center in New York and then the Branch Davidian standoff in Waco, Texas in the same year.

In the end, the Bureau conceded it failed to develop sufficient evidence to charge Williams with any crime. Williams maintained his innocence throughout the investigation. He had the arrogance to appear on a local television news program proclaiming his innocence of any and all charges of wrongdoing. But finally, Williams could not stand the heat and resigned from Truman.

In January 1994, despite the negative publicity about him and his infamous reputation throughout the healthcare profession, Williams landed a job as director of nursing at Ashland Health Care Center, a nearby nursing home in Missouri.

Didn't the Ashland people read the local news? How could they not have heard of Williams? The death rate at Ashland increased dramatically from the day Williams stepped into his Ashland scrubs. The change was quickly noticed by staff and someone tipped off the Missouri Department of Health and Senior Services about it. By July, they issued a report citing an "abnormal number of deaths." Since Williams was hired, they concluded there were thirty deaths in the home as compared to six the entire previous year. However, an investigation of patient deaths by the local medical examiner once again showed no evidence of foul play, which again shows how difficult it is to stop an MSK in his tracks.

In October of 1995, the VA OIG finally issued its report on the Williams investigation at Truman. They repeated, now for public consumption, that patients were twenty times more likely to die under Williams' care, and most damning, in my opinion, "the dysfunctional top management team at Truman should have alerted law enforcement two months before the FBI was called in." Why weren't they contacted immediately when suspicions arose? I think I knew the answer. It had to do with jurisdiction.

Prosecution of crimes occurring at VA medical centers doesn't automatically fall under the purview of the federal criminal justice system. There are three types of prosecutorial jurisdictions that cover VA medical centers. *Exclusive Jurisdiction* refers to locations considered to be the exclusive territory of the United States where local or state police are excluded from conducting investigations. The VA Medical Center in Northport where Swango worked is an example of such a facility. *Concurrent Jurisdiction* refers to an agreement between the federal and state governments: either the federal or the state criminal justice system can be utilized to prosecute and investigate crimes. An example of this type of jurisdiction can be found at the VA Medical Center in Northampton, Massachusetts, where Kristen Gilbert killed her patients. *Proprietorial Jurisdiction* refers to the rarest of the three. In these cases, the state has primary jurisdiction over crimes committed at the VA medical center. This type of jurisdiction covered the Harry S. Truman Medical Center. The problem with proprietorial jurisdiction is that often the local authorities lack the resources to conduct a suspicious death investigation involving numerous victims. This was clearly the case at Truman.

When I talked with a VA attorney about what I might be able to do with Williams, he pointed out to me that the FBI pursued this case as a federal civil rights violation of wrongful death. This offense, unlike murder, has a five-year statute of limitations. After that time, federal prosecution of this case might not be possible. Well, five years was inching closer and closer, but my interest was to pursue a murder case against Williams. No statute of limitations to worry about there.

So, I had my answer about why local law enforcement was not on the case. They simply did not have the resources and took a back seat to the FBI. I don't blame them.

Quickly following the VA OIG report, the Boone County Medical Examiner, Jay Dix, requested the State Board of Nursing report on deaths at Ashland while Williams worked there. I now had that report along with the tissue samples Dix sent me.

In November 1995, the family of Elzie Havrum, a veteran who died under Williams' care within hours of being admitted to Truman, filed a wrongful death suit against the VA. At the time of the filing, the government had not yet determined the cause of Havrum's death. After more than two years of the pretrial process, the FBI reported in February 1998 that it could not pinpoint the cause of death in the thirteen bodies, including Havrum's, that had been exhumed. The new hospital director, Gary Campbell, famously reacted to the report by saying "this is over with for us."

Nonetheless in July, the civil wrongful death trial began. Medical Examiner Doctor Thomas Young testified that Havrum's death was a homicide caused by codeine poisoning. The federal government disagreed. My friend, Doctor Baden, testified for the government that absent a toxicological finding of poison, it could not be proven that these veterans were murdered. Brian Donnelly, who worked with us on Swango, was one of the FBI toxicologists on this case, along with other federal scientific officials. He was also certain that Doctor Young was mistaken. This was essentially the same conclusion the local district attorney came to when he decided he could not prove a criminal case. Everyone believed Williams was a killer but could not prove it, which is why the government had to defend itself in the civil trial. Reading all the reports convinced me he was guilty of murder, but I understood it could not be proven criminally. However, this was a civil trial where the bar is not set as high as in a criminal case. You *can* convict even if the glove does not fit.

On August 7, 1998, U.S. District Court Judge Nanette Laughrey ruled that in her opinion, there was a preponderance of evidence to show that Havrum was poisoned by Richard Williams. She awarded the family four hundred and fifty thousand dollars.

By the end of the summer of 1998, this case had taken more twists and turns then anyone could possibly have imagined. The OIG issued a report in which it criticized the management of the medical center as being "dysfunctional." Campbell, the new medical center director, considered this entire matter closed. The FBI could not determine the cause of death. The statute of limitations on the federal civil rights case had just about ended. And if that wasn't bad enough, now it was time for congressional critics and the media to mount their assault.

An ABC *Primetime Live* episode detailing the Williams civil case was broadcast on January 7, 1998. During the episode, Iowa Senator Charles Grassley, during a congressional hearing on the case, said, "This case was botched from the very beginning by everyone, not just the FBI." The senator was then seen questioning FBI Director Louis Freeh. Freeh appeared incapable of answering the senator's questions but promised to get back to him with answers. In the very next scene, Grassley charged Freeh with failing to get back to him about the case and called Freeh a liar. There were many other media stories just as critical of the VA and FBI in this case. The following year, Christensen, among others, testified before Congress about the harassment and poor treatment he and his colleagues received from the Truman VA Hospital management when they tried to blow the whistle on Williams' alleged murderous ways.

By the time I got the files on the case, there were two congressional hearings that lambasted both the VA and the FBI—a civil trial in which a federal judge stated that in her opinion, Williams did murder a veteran, and a series of toxicological tests that had already failed to identify the cause of death. I understood why Griffin thought it might be better off just letting the matter fade away. That was certainly the opinion of one of my former supervisors as well as the opinion of my counterpart in Chicago whose jurisdiction covered

Truman. He argued that the VA medical center was just recovering from the bad publicity surrounding this case and reopening this matter would set them back years in terms of public relations.

CHAPTER 19

New Evidence!

"Three things cannot be long hidden:
the sun, the moon, and the truth."

—BUDDHA

I called on the same team of Bruce's Angels that performed so brilliantly on Swango to join me in the Big Apple. I needed them to begin their review of the records I had already gone over concerning the Williams investigation. Within a week, the team agreed many of the patients might have died as a result of a phenomenon known as electromechanical disassociation (EMD). They describe it this way:

> The heart muscle contracts (beats) as a result of electrical impulses that travel down special electrical conducting pathways, much like wires going to an electric water pump. This is truly electrical activity and can be measured in mili-amps. For the whole system to function properly, there must first be the electrical impulse, then the heart muscle must be capable of responding to that stimulation by squeezing and pumping blood. In

177

EMD, the electrical impulse and conduction are okay, but the heart can't respond to it by pumping blood. So what you see is an EKG (which is just a graph of the heart's electrical activity) that may look fine, but there is no response by the heart (that is, no pumping of blood and no palpable pulse).

In the water Pump Analogy, *The Wires Are Hot But The Pump Is Broke.* Doctors call it Pulseless Electric Activity.

The nurses concluded that death may have been brought on by the administration of a drug that paralyzed the patients' ability to breathe on their own. There was one such drug available to nurse Richard Williams, succinylcholine, one of the drugs weaponized by Swango. That was something we knew about but because Swango pleaded guilty; we never had to prove that he had used this particular drug in a court of law. Swango admitted in open court only to using a paralytic without naming it. I wished now that the judge would have asked him to be specific. It would have made the job in front of us much easier.

Regarding Williams, it would be incumbent upon us to use the science provided by my team to prove with certainty that succinylcholine was used to kill the Truman veterans. We had one step up on the process; the tissue samples that were retained from the original exhumations and autopsies were available and could be retested. Thankfully, since 1992, when the first tests were performed, science had greatly improved so that a new testing process was available. My team was certain it would be reliable enough to be accepted by the courts.

National Medical Services (NMS), a private lab located outside of Philadelphia, Pennsylvania, had in fact just successfully utilized the new test at the trial of Doctor William Sybers, a medical examiner accused of killing his wife. The inventor of this test was Doctor Kevin Ballard of NMS. In 1999, prosecutors discovered what they believed was the true murder weapon in that case, a chemical injected into Kay Sybers' body, succinylmonocholine. It was a derivative of the muscle relaxant succinylcholine, or "suc," used in surgery, with which we were very familiar. The chemical does not occur naturally in the body and usually dissolves quickly. The prosecutor in the Sybers case said it had been preserved, rather than erased, by the embalming process. "Succinylmonocholine could not be in Kay Sybers' body but through murder," he successfully argued. Doctor Sybers was found guilty of injecting his wife with this deadly chemical.

When I brought this to IG Griffin's attention, he agreed to fund the testing of the tissues in the Williams case in the same manner. The search for the poison had begun.

Doctor Ballard and the people at NMS lived on the cutting edge of the science of toxicology. That made them a target for challenges. I never liked the term "junk science" but even a first-year law student knows some defense attorney would use it as a hammer to smash a prosecutor's case.

Personal injury lawyers often are accused of using highly controversial scientific tests to bamboozle juries into awarding large verdicts. Even government regulators have been accused of utilizing junk science to increase the size of their budgets. Individual scientists may use it to achieve fame and fortune.

The federal courts have placed a considerable burden of proof on the government before it can introduce new science into the courtroom. On occasion, verdicts have been overturned because the "new scientific test" the government relied on proved to be unreliable and riddled with problems. By building a case against Williams based on NMS discovery of "suc" in the bodies of the victims—which caused paralysis, stoppage of the heart, and death—we were walking a path that could be a minefield of challenges.

During the Gilbert case, NMS revealed to the government certain mistakes it had made during its analyses of tissues in search of a deadly drug. It was our duty to reveal them even though they were not identified by the defense. The government correctly withdrew this science from the case. That was not a case of "junk science," but merely a case of an honest error that developed during the scientific process that was immediately disclosed to the court.

On May 16, 2002, NMS reported that succinylmonocholine was present in tissue samples from ten of the thirteen patients whose bodies were exhumed in 1993. Two weeks later, the Boone County Medical Examiner changed the death certificates on these ten individuals to read "homicide." On June 3, 2002, Kevin Crane, the Boone County district attorney, charged Williams with ten counts of first-degree murder. Wayne Kessler, the VA OIG special agent working this case, accompanied by local police, arrested Williams. The alleged killer acted surprised and said the officers were wasting their time. Kessler replied, "I have one word for you: succinylcholine."

The prosecution team was confident it could win a conviction at trial based on the circumstantial evidence. There were no witnesses who could say they saw Williams inject "suc" into a patient. But by following the Red Flags Protocol, the circumstantial evidence was powerful. He worked alone on the ward during the midnight shift, he had access to the suc, he was the last person to see the victims alive, and he showed no remorse. While Williams sat in jail without bail for a year, we prepared for the case. Then things started to fall apart in rapid succession.

First, the Florida appeals court ruled that the toxicology used by NMS and verified by the FBI to find succinylcholine in the Sybers case was not reliable enough to justify a conviction in a Florida court; they ordered a new trial. In order to avoid another trial, Doctor Sybers pleaded guilty in May 2003 to manslaughter, was sentenced to probation, and had to pay three hundred and fifty thousand dollars in investigative costs to the State. Although this development could prove problematic, DA Crane still felt confident about a guilty verdict for Williams. That confidence was shattered when he received the results of the FBI lab report that were issued in an attempt to corroborate the findings of NMS. The FBI report indicated that not only did they find succinylmonocholine in the veterans, they also found it in all the control tissues they tested as well. Those samples should not have had any of this chemical in it. In fact, utilizing NMS' test, succinylmonocholine was found in a calf's liver as well. The NMS test was now considered unreliable. Prosecutor Crane felt he now had no choice but to dismiss the charges against Williams, despite the strong circumstantial case. If we could not be certain there was "suc" in the bodies, the circumstances did not matter.

I was not to have my day in court against Williams. It was a terrible disappointment, especially since I had argued so strenuously with Griffin to let me expend resources going after Williams again. My team—Bruce's Angels, the agents on the case, the scientists and technicians, Baden, Rieders, and Ballard—all experienced an overwhelming sense of frustration. I did not doubt my actions for one second. It was my duty to go after a man I believed was a killer. But he had escaped the hangman's noose.

The most painful part was informing the families that the case had gone to hell. Most of them took the news with grace and thanked us for trying. Some could not understand the legal system at work. No one doubted Williams was an MSK who would go free.

At a news conference discussing his decision to release Williams, Crane said he still felt that Williams was guilty but could not pursue the case given the lack of toxicological evidence. Williams made a bizarre statement on his own behalf: *I would have to say, given the erroneous data Mr. Crane had, the charges were appropriate.*

To me, they were the words of someone who was still in shock that he beat the rap for a crime he had actually committed. A victim's family member told the local media, "It looks like he got away with murder."

While attending a meeting of the American Academy of Forensic Sciences in February 2004, I learned that Richard Williams had filed a lawsuit against National Medical Services and Doctor Ballard, claiming that their bogus scientific conclusions caused his incarceration and suffering as a result. The man I believed responsible for the death of at least ten of our nation's veterans was trying to profit from his actions. Fortunately, all courts that heard this claim dismissed it and Williams has not collected a dime.

Williams remains an enigmatic figure in the law enforcement community. From time to time rumors surface that range from the killing of his two children and his mother, to his work in a fast food restaurant in the Midwest. But, I don't know for sure.

CHAPTER 20

What Makes Them Tick?

*"Destroy the seed of evil, or it will grow up to your
ruin."*

—AESOP

The entire episode with Williams—starting from when I first
heard about him from IG Griffin to the day when he beat
the rap for the second time—left me stunned and bewildered.
Never before had I been involved in such a disturbing case. Of
course, not every suspect I arrested in my twenty-plus-year career up until that point was convicted and sent to prison, but
until I met Michael Swango, those were criminals of a different
type. They were con artists, thieves, drug dealers, embezzlers, an
occasional sexual predator. But until my encounter with "Double O Swango" they were not homicidal maniacs. I understood
what made them tick: it was usually greed, a profit motive, or
some sexual impulse that made them take advantage of a patient, coworker, or the government.

With the MSKs, there was something darker, more deeply embedded in their consciousness that I could not possibly

wrap my hands around. Swango liked to watch people slowly slip into a coma-like state, then expire. He would sit and stare at the patient and the network of streaming graphs, flashing lights, and beeping tones that indicted the very state of the patient's life. When all signs indicated death, Swango's personal mission was accomplished.

Gilbert's thrill was in the glory she received as she rushed to "save" a patient's life. Did she recognize that she was the person who caused the patient to be in distress? What was she thinking? Was she a sociopath?

And what was Williams? The allegations against him were the most heinous I ever heard. In my mind, I did not even visualize Williams as human. To me, he was some other-worldly being without shape or form. But Williams was never convicted of a murder. How could I be so wrong? What was going through his mind when the charges against him were dropped? Did he breathe a sigh of relief? Did he actually believe he was innocent? What made him tick?

Those were the hardest questions to answer.

In 2005, shortly after I retired from the VA and opened my own private investigations firm, I attended an FBI Serial Murder Symposium in San Antonio, Texas. There were many psychologists, homicide detectives, and agents from the Bureau's Behavioral Analysis Unit (BAU) in attendance. I knew some of them and made it a point to meet others. I wanted to hear their views on the question that was bothering me. I understood the Red Flags Protocol explained behavior that could identify and stop an MSK but before it could be effective, the suspect had to have established a pattern of behavior, such as involvement in an unusual amount of code incidents. But if we knew what made them tick, perhaps they could be stopped before they got a job in the healthcare profession.

It was in San Antonio that I first heard the phrase, "Munchausen's Syndrome" as a possible explanation. The name comes from Baron von Munchausen, a colorful 18th century figure known for wild fabrications about his travels and exploits. In 1951, the term "Munchausen Syndrome" was first used by the medical profession to describe patients who invented symptoms, so they could subject themselves to frequent medical procedures. Longtime VA healthcare professionals know the legend of "Major Munchausen," a World War II veteran who traveled across the country visiting VA hospitals in order to receive treatment for various illnesses. Trouble was he never actually had those illnesses. His MO was to study the symptoms of a particular illness so he could carefully and accurately explain to the doctors what he was experiencing, that he was suffering, and that he needed help.

Of course, the doctors realized that the "Major" was bizarrely fabricating his distress to get their attention. When the doctors revealed they were on to his game and suggested he might want to accept psychiatric care. he would act insulted and stomp out of the facility, eager to move on to the next VA hospital. His behavior wasn't really affecting anyone other than taking up valuable doctors' time and he was usually dealt with compassionately.

The "by proxy" condition refers to inventing or inducing sickness in another, as when a mother brings her child to an emergency room claiming falsely the youngster has one disease or another in order to bring attention to herself as a caring mother. Or, when by being a hero during a code, a medical professional brings attention to herself by displaying her considerable skills and talents. That was certainly a pattern of behavior in Gilbert and somewhat in Swango.

But what of the medical professionals who kill simply because they don't like a certain patient, are too lazy to continue care for a difficult patient, or those who sincerely believe they want to end the victim's suffering. That was what the New Jersey nurse, Charles Cullen, claimed. After he was arrested, he said he had no desire to fight any charges brought against him and that he had killed as many as forty patients to end their suffering. Looking back on that case with the knowledge I have gained, I don't believe Cullen gave a damn about the suffering of patients. He was a seriously ill person, discharged from the Navy after suicide attempts, and should never have been allowed near patients.

The infamous record on MSKs reveals these killers are encouraged by the fact that they can easily continue to kill, sometimes for years, without suspicion. Once suspicion arises, they simply move on to the next medical institution with a good or at worst neutral recommendation and continue to kill unabated. Some killers grow to believe that they possess some special power or divine right to kill patients since they continue to be successful for such a long period of time.

In a 1991 interview with a reporter from the the *Columbus Dispatch in Ohio*, VA nurse Donald Harvey, who claimed to have murdered eighty-seven people, was asked: "Why did you kill?" His answer: "Well, people controlled me for eighteen years, and then I controlled my own destiny. I controlled other people's lives; whether they lived or died, I had that power to control."

"What right did you have to decide that?" the reporter asked.

"After I didn't get caught for the first fifteen, I thought it was my right. I appointed myself judge, prosecutor, and jury. So I played God."

I have yet to come across a doctor or scientist who can explain exactly why serial killers do what they do. Some say it might be in their DNA. Some point to the upbringing of the killer; cruel, abusive parents are often heard of as part of a defense for a killer on trial. A domineering, former soldier raised Swango, Gilbert seems to have come from a troubled home, and Cullen was raped by his father. But did that turn them into MSKs? No one really knows. The greatest common denominator it seems is the obsession with being in control. What greater level of control is there than the power of life and death?

I first learned of MSKs while working for the VA. I admit to wondering if these monsters intentionally chose the VA over other medical institutions. Over the years, I have not seen evidence indicating that serial killers intentionally targeted the VA. There have been plenty of hospital serial killers in the private sector throughout history. But it sticks in my mind that a VA medical center is a perfect hunting ground. The VA facilities are filled with long-term care patients with serious debilitating illnesses. Family members rarely if ever visit them at the medical center.

A related thought of mine, a thought I cannot shake, is whether serial killers intentionally choose the medical profession? What comes first, the chicken or the egg? Does the killer choose the hunting ground or does the hunting ground seduce the potential killer? I have not found evidence to support either answer. But if I were a serial killer looking for a profession where I could get away with murder, the medical field would be high on my list. These are professions where the victims and their families put their implicit trust in caregivers. It is an environment where death is a common occurrence and can be attributed to either natural causes or medical error. It has been estimated that more than ninety thousand patients die as the result of medical errors in hospitals each year in the United States.

It is also an environment that is unfamiliar territory to police; they don't understand the terminology, the policies and procedures, or the recordkeeping system. A killer can arrange to work alone at night and have the authority to draw a curtain around a potential victim, only then to sit and watch the victim die.

There is never a need to smuggle in a gun or a knife into the killing ground. There are many death-dealing untraceable chemicals available. The attack does not leave stab wounds, bullet holes, or contusions; it is as easy as inserting a poison-filled syringe into an existing line or tube. Even if the victim cries out when a doctor or nurse tries to kill him, probably no one will pay any attention because those cries are common on the wards of a hospital or nursing home. If the victim continues to complain, staff may note in his file he suffers from some psychological ailment because he thought his doctor or nurse was trying to kill him. Lastly, even if someone suspects foul play, management will bend over backwards to defend a suspected killer and prove that the victim died of natural causes. In a worst-case scenario, management may ask for a suspect's resignation, but they will likely provide a positive letter of recommendation, smoothing a path to the next facility where killing can begin again. Unfortunately, these cynical comments are a result of years of investigating MSKs and developing an insight into how they operate.

There is another side to this coin I think of when I sometimes get down on our medical profession. It is important to remember that while hospitals provide an easy killing ground for MSKs, providing the opportunities, weapons, and means for escape, they also represent a place of compassion, brilliance, and often lifesaving miracles.

I read a newspaper story written by William L. Solomon, a veteran of the World War II Okinawa campaign, that comes to mind whenever I am too immersed in the evil world of MSKs for my own good.

The story is about a medical professional who had intentions of killing, but whose training, professionalism, and human nature quickly dissuaded him from the act. "The Combat Medic" appeared in the March 6, 2001, edition of Long Island's *Newsday*. Solomon reports he once felt that if he ever had the chance to get a Japanese soldier at the business end of a hypodermic needle, he would inject the enemy with some poison-like arsenic. He was assigned to a hospital that treated Japanese prisoners of war and one day his chance came.

> "But when I went into the hospital ward, I was struck by the sight of the wounded, the stench of gangrene and rot, the cries of pain. The gloomy lantern light made me feel that I was back somewhere in the pre-historic days. My hatred melted. These people could not hurt me— they were on their backs. I realized, after the first few hours on that job that I wasn't going to kill anybody. I realized that these people were weak and helpless. You could never tell who the enemy was on Okinawa, but, enemy or not, I felt sorry for one of the wounded women who, after thanking me for my aid, died in my arms. Hatred is a strong feeling, a powerful word, but there are stronger feelings than hatred. Sometimes one particular feeling will conquer hatred. That feeling is not just sympathy—it's a sense of fair play."

The overwhelming majority of medical professionals throughout the world exhibit this sense of fair play, sympathy, and compassion every minute of every day. This is the other side of the coin.

CHAPTER 21

The Survambulance

"Bruce, this is a violation of the Geneva Convention."

—DOCTOR MICHAEL BADEN

While I was becoming more and more caught up in the world of MSKs, it concerned me that I was losing sight of other things that were going on. I needed a good case to regain my focus, and to no one's surprise, there was some action at Northport that needed my attention.

Any institution that has pharmaceuticals, narcotics, and a patient population of drug addicts and drug-seeking patients will inevitably experience illegal drug dealing in its facility. It is a problem common to public and private hospitals alike. VA hospitals are no exception. Patients are known to sell their drugs right on the grounds of the VA medical centers or methadone maintenance clinics nearby. The dealers and users with VA property mirrored the same scene taking place on the streets. The patients, staff, and visitors doing this are criminals. And they become as adept at avoiding the law as

191

any of their brethren out on the streets and parking lots of Anytown, USA.

They quickly expose undercover agents, they get wise to patient informants, and they use intimidation and violence to enforce the rules of their illicit business. Over the years, the VA police, my colleagues in the IG offices around the country, the FBI, and the DEA—have collaborated on successful task forces and operations to bring networks of dealers down in order to clean up facilities. Unfortunately, they come back, just like out in the real world.

I was dismayed by the fact that brave veterans came home from war not only with physical wounds, but also with addiction to drugs that would surely kill them if not brought under control. I was always anxious to have my office cooperate in local police operations that touched on VA employees and facilities. In the mid-1990s, I created a special drug unit that was cross-designated with the DEA, thus enabling full participation in ongoing tactical operations.

We took part in several long-term projects. One in Clarksburg, West Virginia, stands out as an example of how sophisticated cooperation can have dynamic results.

We called it "Operation Protect the Vet." It was a joint effort of local, state, and federal investigators, and in July of 2003, we arrested fourteen dealers who were operating near a VA facility. Included in the task force was an undercover agent, who managed to survive more than a year working within the dealers' gangs to provide vital information to us.

The gangs operated a private club they called "The Veterans Club" about two blocks from the medical center. Their main business was selling crack cocaine to veterans, but they also traded in drugs stolen from the VA pharmacy or prescribed to the vets, who would give them up for money.

After we brought the club and dealers down, I was encouraged to ask my bosses in DC for permission to expand my special cross-designated unit. However, I was stopped dead in my tracks by the IG counsel, who argued that we were prohibited by statute from financing any IG/police hybrid team, no matter how honorable our intentions. Rather than find a way to work with these outside law enforcement groups as many of the VA medical center directors wanted, we were forced to disband the special unit by red tape that no one wanted to even try to cut. My reputation as an aggressive supervisor had grown impressively since Swango but I can't say it made friends for me throughout the VA system. The counsel was always looking over my shoulder. Well, I guess that was her job, as mine was to look over the shoulders of thousands of VA employees. At the end of the day, I thought service to our veterans was our driving force.

Working with just my unit. I managed to tackle that drug problem at Northport in a manner that has become part of VA lore.

There was a preschool facility at Northport and the area outside had become a meeting place for users and dealers to do their business. Vets who were in a methadone program would pick up their supply, then head directly to that area to either sell it or trade it for cocaine. We had a terrific African-American undercover agent loaned to us by the VA police in DC who was able to identify all the leaders among the dealers. He was so good at blending in with them that we sometimes worried he would get caught up in a raid by the local police in town.

One element of the case we were building against these drug dealers was photos of them in action. We wanted to capture shots of our agents buying drugs and we wanted to prove they did business within one thousand feet of the preschool, which would increase the penalties against them.

That presented a problem for us because we did not have a place to hide the camera and recording equipment. We had a couple of nondescript vehicles in our fleet of government vehicles, but like surveillance vehicles manufactured for law enforcement, they had a certain look to them that streetsmart characters picked up in an instant. They were usually white vans with a vent on the top that was actually used for surveillance. They could cost more than one hundred thousand dollars brand-new, and were equipped with cameras, recording devices, and other surveillance items. I can tell you from experience that sitting on a hot day in one of those units with the engine off and no air conditioning, was close to unbearable.

So, if an agent were sitting in a white unmarked van with the engine running in the summer with darkened windows, the chances were it was a surveillance van and the police were inside watching. But my A team, as usual, came through with a solution that is still talked about in agent school. What kind of vehicle could remain running while sitting in one place on the grounds of a hospital for a long period of time without drawing suspicion? An ambulance, of course! And we found one in the Northport fleet that suited our needs. It had a lot of years and miles on it and plenty of dents and dings. I have to admit that when I first saw it, I thought I could whip it into shape like I did in my garage with my old Buicks. I would have gladly taken a crack at it but we agreed it looked more "real" with its age showing. Anyway, we had a guy who could make everything work.

George Blydenburgh was a VA biomedical engineer and electronic genius. Around headquarters we called him "Q" like the James Bond character who created all the life-saving gadgets 007 used to get out of jams. George made all the mechanical repairs needed and placed cameras and recording devices all around the vehicle. It all cost less than twenty thousand dollars. We called the unit "survambulance"—part ambulance and part surveillance vehicle.

It was an immediate success when we parked it near the preschool. Not only were our perpetrators unable to identify the vehicle, they actually conducted hundreds of illicit drug sales standing right outside the front windows of the survambulance. From time to time we would move the unit, turning on the lights and sirens and speeding off to an unknown destination, then returning in a few minutes, just to establish its legitimacy. But that was probably not even necessary. These dealers were so arrogant and confident no one was watching them that they were stunned when we lowered the boom and put about a dozen in handcuffs.

One night at dinner, I told my friend Doctor Baden about the success of the survambulance and he responded with a chuckle, "Bruce, this is a violation of the Geneva Convention."

The IG was so impressed by the operation he suggested we re-create our vehicle and sell them at a profit to other agencies. Well, we never did that but we sure caught a lot of bad guys who were shocked to learn that the ambulance was really the survambulance. Only instead of taking sick people to the hospital, it was taking bad guys off the street.

CHAPTER 22

Prosecution Declined

*"Keep away from small people who try to belittle
your ambitions. Small people always do that, but the
really great make you feel that you, too, can become
great."*

—MARK TWAIN

The Williams case did not conclude with the outcome I
hoped and worked hard for, but I was satisfied that we all
did our jobs honestly and correctly. From my lowest-ranking
agents to the nurses and to the US Attorneys involved, we all
stayed on the same page and pursued a difficult goal.

I can't say the same about a case in New England in which
I believe a US Attorney failed to have the courage to do the
right thing despite the concentration of evidence my team
brought to the table. In fairness, I have changed the name
of the suspect and the facility in question but here is how I
remember it.

At the Federal Law Enforcement Training Center, I once
taught a course titled, Presenting Cases to US Attorneys. I
instructed young agents attending the Inspector General

training program to proceed very carefully before deciding to appeal a decision to decline prosecution of a case by a local US Attorney to a higher authority. Not only would the request more than likely be denied, but the local US Attorney's Office would despise you for taking that step and find a way to retaliate. However, the case of Doctor Richard Sheldon forced me to go against my own teachings and appeal a decision from the US Attorney The result was unfortunately exactly similar to what I consistently preached.

A patient at the Bernard VA Medical Center in New England had been placed on a "comfort measures only" (CMO) regime. It is a protocol designed for patients that have terminal illnesses and for whom a Do Not Resuscitate Order (DNR) is already in place. The comfort of the patient is the primary goal when he or she is in a terminal stage. The medical committees that design these procedures make it abundantly clear that assisting someone in this regard clearly does not mean accelerating the patient's demise for any reason. Yet, in my opinion, VA physician Sheldon took it upon himself to do just that and then bragged about it to his staff. When I heard about this, I thought he should pay a penalty for that violation of morality, medical ethics, and civil law. I thought he was guilty of murder.

Doctor Sheldon was the chief surgical resident at Bernard at the time a terminally ill veteran was treated in the ICU when on a Sunday in March, he was transferred to Doctor Sheldon's unit.

On the following morning, Doctor Sheldon requested a nurse to administer a dose of morphine in excess of seventy-five mg to the patient. Believing the dose was so high it would kill the patient, the nurse refused the doctor's request.

Doctor Sheldon then performed the procedure himself. The process involved flushing the contents of an intravenous storage bag through an infusion pump that was attached to the veteran. The patient died within minutes of receiving the dose of morphine.

It was learned that Doctor Sheldon acknowledged to members of his unit that morning that he had administered the fatal dose of morphine. He said he knew the quantity was large, and that he wanted the veteran to die. Sheldon had also stated that the veteran had been CMO since the previous Friday, three days earlier, and that the family wanted the veteran to die. He explained it was up to him to put the veteran's wife out of her misery. Doctor Sheldon told colleagues the patient was going to die anyway, and all he did was hasten it along. He took full responsibility, according to witnesses. To the credit of the management of this VA medical center, the US Attorney's Office was promptly notified, and my office was brought in on a joint investigation. I quickly got VA OIG Special Agent Jack Leonard on the case, and soon we were working again with the brilliant FBI Special Agent Brian Donnelly.

Leonard soon gathered all the available physical evidence that would be useful to the government prosecuting the case and began interviewing witnesses who relayed the conversations about Sheldon's admissions regarding the injection and his motive.

Donnelly sent the infusion pump to the manufacturer for testing. It was found to be functioning properly. Raw data collected from the pump event history log showed that the pump flow setting had been increased several times to allow the content of the intravenous bag to flow more freely through the pump. The only reason for this was that someone was turning the pump into a murder weapon.

The local medical examiner performed the autopsy. The report listed the cause of death as acute morphine overdose, the manner of death as homicide, and the circumstances of death as "administration of morphine in excess of comfort measures only advanced directives." This meant that the patient died not from any natural disease processes, but from the administration of an overdose of morphine. So, the medical examiner believed the patient died as a result of human action, but "homicide" does not necessarily mean "murder," which is a criminal act.

We brought in a medical ethicist from Harvard University to review the facts of the case. He concurred that Doctor Sheldon's actions were illegal and unethical.

I thought we buttoned the case up really well. We had witnesses who saw Doctor Sheldon administer the morphine, a nurse that declined to follow his order to do the same because she thought it was a fatal dose, and several individuals ready to testify that he admitted to what he had done. Backing up our total theory of murder was the deceased veteran's family, who vehemently denied ever asking Doctor Sheldon to end their loved one's life. I was confident we would easily convince the US Attorney to seek a murder indictment.

Boy was I wrong.

Despite the facts I presented, the US Attorney's Office saw things differently. Its opinion was the veteran was near death, was about to expire imminently anyway, and that it would be too difficult to prove a criminal charge against Sheldon, especially a murder charge. They rejected the medical examiner's opinion as being based on a legal standard less than their own for prosecution decisions.

Margaret Curran, the US Attorney, wrote to me in a letter, "As you may be aware, the legal standard for the medical examiner's finding is probable cause. The same standard applies to a grand jury's determination that criminal charges ought to be filed. Our prosecutive decisions, however, are guided by a much higher standard."

She was wrong. The legal standard for the medical examiner's findings is not probable cause. The standard is reasonable degree of medical and scientific certainty. What I took from the letter was that Curran was not convinced she could unquestionably win a conviction. Therefore, she declined the case. I thought that was a dereliction of duty.

Under that guideline, some of the greatest cases in American history would have never been prosecuted. In my opinion, her argument was ill-conceived, and quite frankly her decision to decline prosecution was cowardly. I felt strongly that Sheldon did not simply ease a patient into a peaceful death,but had decided to play God and end the life of the veteran at his own time and choosing.

I called a meeting with attorneys from the Justice Department and the US Attorney's Office, including Ms. Curran, to argue that she change her mind and call for prosecution. I enlisted my trusted allies—Doctor Michael Baden, Brian Donnelly, Jack Leonard, and a few others to be on my side. Although the meeting became quite argumentative at times, as everyone said their piece, our argument fell on deaf ears. Curran would not budge from her decision not to pursue the case.

So here is where I decided to go against my own teachings to my new agents. I took the unusual step of appealing the US Attorney's decision to the US Department of Justice in

Washington, D.C., the office that is commonly referred to as "Main Justice."

The attorneys from Main Justice, after considering the matter for some time, decided not to overrule the US Attorney's decision even though they basically agreed with many of our arguments. This was politics. The Department of Justice (DOJ) sided with the US Attorney against the VA. I saw it no other way. There was no other rational explanation. I felt this entire exercise was a colossal waste of time and a dereliction of justice for this vet and his family.

Not long after that meeting at Main Justice, it was widely reported in the news media that the widow of the veteran was suing the VA and Doctor Sheldon separately for a total of twenty million dollars. To me that was further validation that Doctor Sheldon was lying when he said the family wanted him to end the veteran's life ASAP. If they wanted him to die, they sure had a funny way of expressing their appreciation with a twenty million dollar lawsuit.

The lawsuit against the VA was settled for seven hundred and fifty thousand dollars. And the family dropped its suit against Sheldon.

I tell this story to my students as an example. I believe the DOJ and US Attorney stood up against the VA. So, as I said, I caution my agents to avoid appealing a decision that might go against them. However, I also tell them that our job is to seek justice and that is not something that should be abandoned easily, without a fight.

CHAPTER 23

Research Murder...

"Research is what I'm doing when I don't know what
I'm doing."

—WERNHER VON BRAUN

Throughout history, great strides in the field of medicine have been the result of incredible research done by dedicated scientists focused on improving the lives of people. Much of this research is conducted in hospitals funded in large part by government money acquired through the process of grants. This is true in all the great private and public hospitals, including VA facilities. It is impossible to count the number of lives saved as a result of this research, which costs more than a billion dollars a year. In a typical year, the VA may conduct fifteen thousand studies using one hundred and fifty thousand veteran-patients, with a large portion coming from the private sector.

I take great pride in the VA's role in medical research. VA doctors and scientists were responsible for such medical breakthroughs as the first implantable cardiac pacemaker, the first successful liver transplants, the nicotine patch, and therapies to help smokers give up the habit. In fact, the reason why many of us take one aspirin a day, to reduce the risk of heart attack, was demonstrated during VA studies. Today, the VA leads the way in the development of prostheses used to treat veterans grievously wounded in combat. These are but a few examples of notable achievements.

Besides grants, money comes from other government agencies, nonprofit organizations, and for-profit pharmaceutical companies. VA researchers, however, are not compensated directly from the pharmaceutical companies. The VA cannot accept money directly from outside sources. So, Congress authorized the VA to establish nonprofit research corporations that are allowed to accept private funding, and retain a portion for overhead and general and administrative expenses. The remainder of the money is placed in a designated account as a research budget for VA medical investigators who receive research funding.

This money cannot be used to supplement the salary of the researcher, but can be used for all other expenses pertaining to the research project including salaries of staff, necessary supplies, travel to conferences, laboratory equipment, and so on. Quite an empire can be built through medical research monies. At times, some VA researchers may be involved in so many projects that, finding themselves overextended, that they begin to take shortcuts. Sometimes the consequences of those shortcuts are devastating.

Medical history is filled with examples of research that today we find barbaric and inhumane. During the Middle Ages doctors, using condemned prisoners, would purposely inflict a combat-type wound on the hapless subject in order to judge whether it would be fatal and, if not, to try to figure the best way to treat it. As gruesome as it sounds, it undoubtedly led to advances in treating wounds caused by the most primitive of weapons like lances, spears, and heavy chains.

Nazi doctors infamously experimented on live concentration camp inmates in order to achieve such medical outcomes as improving survival in freezing water for downed pilots and finding treatment for infections that they inflicted. Some of those doctors were madmen and were punished as war criminals.

Richard Williams may have been the case that most frustrated me in my pursuit of MSKs but the case of Paul Kornak was the one that creeped me out more than any other. Kornak offered hope to veterans seriously ill with different kinds of cancer, then duped them into taking part in an experimental process for which they were not medically qualified. He falsified reports to get them into experimental chemotherapy programs in order to keep the flow of money from the pharmaceutical companies funding the programs. He needed subjects and that is all that mattered to him.

I was not surprised there was trouble at the Stratton VA Medical Center in Albany, New York. The facility had a terrible reputation for sloppiness, especially in the research department, and there were consistent rumblings among the rank and file that risked the careers of whistleblowers if they came forward. But I had never been called in to take a look at anything up there.

The Albany Research Institute (ARI), a nonprofit corporation, was established to handle funding for research conducted at Stratton. On January 11, 1999, Kornak was hired by ARI to conduct data coordination and monitoring of ongoing cancer studies. His title was program specialist and his starting salary was 61,836 dollars. As I began my investigation, I was quickly thunderstruck by a similarity between Kornak and Swango. They were both natural-born, lying, con artists.

A routine audit of Kornak's project turned up accounting discrepancies. That report landed on my desk. All the problems led me to Kornak, so I took a look at his file.

Once again, I was embarrassed by the incomprehensible laxity of the administrative bosses at a VA medical center. Did they not understand the meaning of the words "background check?"

I easily turned up information on Kornak. The furthest he went in school was completion of his undergraduate studies at the Junior College of Albany and the College of Saint Rose, both in New York State.

However, he applied for his medical license in New Jersey. He made his application to the New Jersey Board of Medical Examiners in September 1989. With his application to the board, Kornak submitted fraudulent transcripts from those two schools in which he made extensive alterations. He added courses that he had not taken, he raised many of the grades that he received, and he changed his actual cumulative averages to reflect those alterations. He stamped the word "OFFICIAL" on the fraudulent transcripts and dated them to reflect a date later than when he actually attended those schools.

In addition, he submitted transcripts from the Wroclaw Medical University in Poland. These were totally false documents, which he created. This reminded me of Swango's creation of a fictitious letter from a governor that supposedly restored his civil rights and helped him get a position at Stony Brook University Hospital. However, the investigative record shows that "transcripts" from Poland, as well as

Kornak's altered undergraduate transcripts, were accepted by St. George's University School of Medicine in Grenada, and Ross University School of Medicine in, Dominica. In his New Jersey testimony to the board, Kornak said he was enrolled at St. George's for approximately eighteen months and left because he could not pay his tuition. In actuality, he was dismissed from St. George's University for altering a transcript and sending it to a potential employer, Highland Hospital in Rochester, New York.

The New Jersey Board of Medical Examiners found that Kornak had falsified many of the documents that he had filed with his application for licensing in New Jersey. The board found that his testimony before the credential committee was unreliable and contradictory, and that he had been untruthful in many particulars. The board further resolved to refer the matter to St. George's University and Ross University.

In July 1990, he was denied a license to practice medicine in New Jersey. At least the New Jersey Board of Examiners knew how to conduct a background check. Nonetheless, Kornak proceeded to identify himself as an MD as he looked for work in the metropolitan area.

Amazingly, Kornak had previously obtained medical licenses in Iowa and Pennsylvania. The New Jersey Board of Medical Examiners responsibly forwarded their findings to the Iowa Board of Medicine and the Pennsylvania State Board of Medicine. After reviewing the information, the Iowa Board of Medicine revoked his license on October 7, 1991, and the Pennsylvania State Board of Medicine suspended his license on November 6, 1991.

My initial background check on Kornak also easily turned up the record that Kornak was arrested by US

Postal Inspectors on November 17, 1992, and charged with the federal crime of mail fraud; he falsified the records he had sent to the Iowa, New Jersey, and Pennsylvania medical boards in an attempt to obtain a valid license to practice medicine in these states. He pleaded guilty, received three years of probation, 200 hours of community service and a two thousand five hundred dollar fine. In spite of a well-documented history of fraud and misrepresentation, seven years later, he was working at Stratton determining which veterans should be placed in life-and-death research studies.

Not long after I was alerted to the problems at Stratton, I learned Kornak was hired in spite of the fact his medical license had been revoked. He allegedly told the chief VA researcher that his license, which had never been awarded in the first place, had been revoked because he could not document his first year of medical school in Poland. No further inquiry about his background was conducted. The laughable explanation I got from the Stratton administration was that detailed background checks were only done on doctors who would be treating patients. Kornak was hired to do research.

I guess they felt that because Kornak had some training as a medical doctor, he would be an excellent research assistant. He certainly possessed more medical education than most other research assistants. A VA researcher could conceivably ask Kornak to perform all sorts of medical analyses a non-physician-trained assistant could never accomplish.

On my first visit up to Stratton, which was about a four-hour drive from New York City, I discovered something deeply disturbing about Kornak's relationship with the VA. One of his colleagues who was suspicious about

Kornak pointed out to me that he wore a hospital ID card that clearly identified him as Paul Kornak, MD. His VA business card identified him the same way. That sort of identification displayed each day on his lab coat would clearly be helpful to him in gaining the trust of patients or family members whose cooperation he needed to continue his experimental chemo treatments.

I began requisitioning more and more paperwork pertaining to Kornak's work. The audit already done was extremely helpful, and at some point, I was making the trek to Stratton a few days a week. Actually, that was the most pleasant part of the investigation. If I did not need the car when I was up there, I would travel by Amtrak from Manhattan's Pennsylvania Station to Albany, a route that hugged the eastern shore of the Hudson River. It was quite beautiful in any season. It was a restful trip allowing me to pore over all those records. One day looking out the window on the frozen Hudson, I realized that Kornak must have had help in his scheme. It was time for me to take a closer look at his supervisors.

For most of the time, he was conducting the chemo experiments, Kornak's immediate supervisor was Doctor James Holland. Holland was a very busy man. He was involved in numerous research projects both inside and outside the VA. In order to complete his current research projects and actively solicit funding for even more, he needed to rely heavily on his research assistants. Kornak, with his extra level of medical expertise, was perfect for Holland. Kornak could operate with less than high supervision and he could help the other researchers while Holland went about the business of keeping the funds flowing. No wonder, I thought, Holland allowed Kornak to pass himself off as an MD. It served Holland's purpose to appeal to Kornak's ego.

I had a strong team of forensic accountants on hand in New York to give me final recommendations regarding any criminal acts that had been committed, but it always helped if I totally understood what they were talking about. Just like when I asked Baden to walk me through an autopsy in progress, I would eventually get the flow of money explained.

I found the process byzantine. I followed the money in a study known as Tax 327, which Holland ran. It involved the testing of a new drug for the treatment of prostate cancer. The agreement between the pharmaceutical company and Holland provided for payment of a maximum of seventy-five thousand dollars on a pro rata basis for ten patients completing the study. Funding would be allocated in stages as patients were enrolled and results were submitted. An amendment on April 25, 2001, increased the number of patients to twenty-five and the maximum payment to one hundred and ninety-two thousand dollars. The site coordinator at the Stratton VAMC was Paul Kornak.

It was clear to me that Kornak's survival as an esteemed researcher, so esteemed, in fact, that he was allowed to pass himself off as an MD, ensured a steady flow of patients into the program. Considering that these patients needed to be suffering from cancer and presumably had been extensively treated already, the challenge for Kornak was to convince them to undergo his experimental treatment.

If he could not locate and enlist a sufficient number of patients for these studies, all funding could be eliminated. If research funding were to be denied, his services would no longer be needed. However, if the research dollars kept flowing, not only would his position be secure but he might be elevated to a higher position in the VA research hierarchy. I learned from their colleagues that Kornak and Holland would fantasize about a new research center being built in Albany that would be run by them. Kornak could certainly help make that a reality if he could maintain their research programs.

In short, patients' records were altered enabling veterans to be enrolled in various research studies for which they were either too sick or too healthy to be eligible. For instance, a patient with coronary disease was enrolled in a study that excluded heart patients over risk of hemorrhages. Another patient with impaired renal function was administered a drug toxic to his kidneys. He died. This was typical of the kind of risks to which Kornak was indifferent.

Families of deceased patients said their loved ones were treated as guinea pigs and that Kornak and Holland were snake oil salesmen offering hope when there was very little hope to offer.

Swango, Gilbert, and even Williams all had some of the con artist in them. They smoothly pulled the wool over the eyes of hospital administrators and obtained positions that should have been denied them based mainly on their prior job performances. And in a way, they conned their victims, who thought they were being cared for while in fact they were being murdered.

Kornak was different. He had to be a supreme con artist as well as a willing killer. He had to convince prospective subjects of the experiments he was conducting to volunteer for the process. He had to look the patients and their wives, daughters or even mothers, in their eyes and say that he held the secret to extending life for their loved ones. What could be creepier than that!

Those loved ones, some who survived the battlefields of Europe and Asia, were losing their personal battles against cancers that were extremely difficult to successfully treat. They clung to any chance of a cure they could find. So, when a smooth-talking con man wearing a white lab coat with an embroidered name and ID that indicated MD approached and informed them what was available, it was difficult not to listen.

The come-on would get even more serious. "By the way," Kornak might say, according to families of deceased vets, "it just so happens that you meet the inclusion criteria to enter this new study." Traditional treatments have been notoriously unsuccessful, but there is a chance, Kornak said, that this study could make a difference. Most of the veterans Kornak approached eagerly jumped at the "opportunity" he was offering. It did not matter that they might have been suffering from cancer of the esophagus and the experimental drug Kornak was testing was for treatment of prostate cancer. It did not matter that a patient did not meet the standards for inclusion. All that could be taken care of by a con artist killer so the drug companies would keep the money flowing.

Human research is the most heavily regulated and audited area in medicine, partly because of the ethical issues involved. There are so many different organizations claiming responsibility for this function that it is difficult to determine who is watching whom. When Kornak was at work, there were at least fifteen government agencies, commissions, or committees, including the Department of Health and Human Services as well as the VA's own Institutional Review Boards, and Site Monitoring, Auditing and Review Teams (SMART), with some level of responsibility for oversight, both ethical and financial. Still, Kornak was able to run his con game. Maybe it was too many cooks in the kitchen.

The more I looked into Kornak, who was fifty-three years old, the more complicated and confusing the case became. I had no doubt there was criminal activity going on. I wasn't sure it reached the level of homicide, but it certainly was more than fraud. I knew I needed to roll out a powerful team of agents to really get to the heart of the matter.

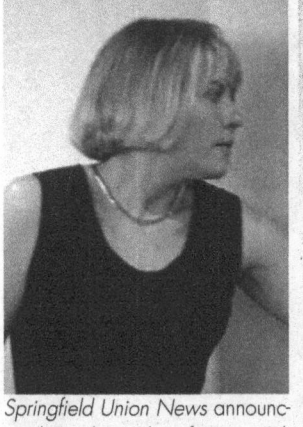

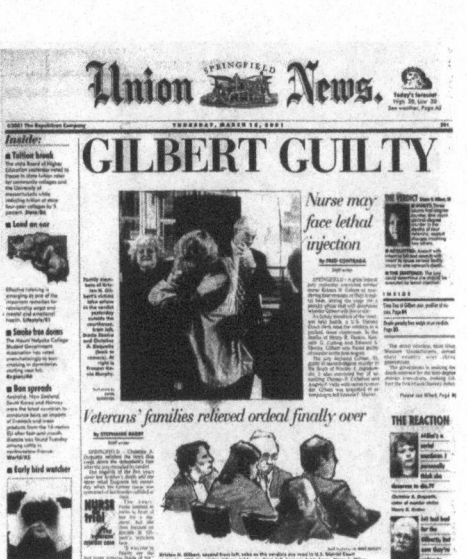

Springfield Union News announcing the guilty verdict of Kristen Gilbert on March 15, 2001.

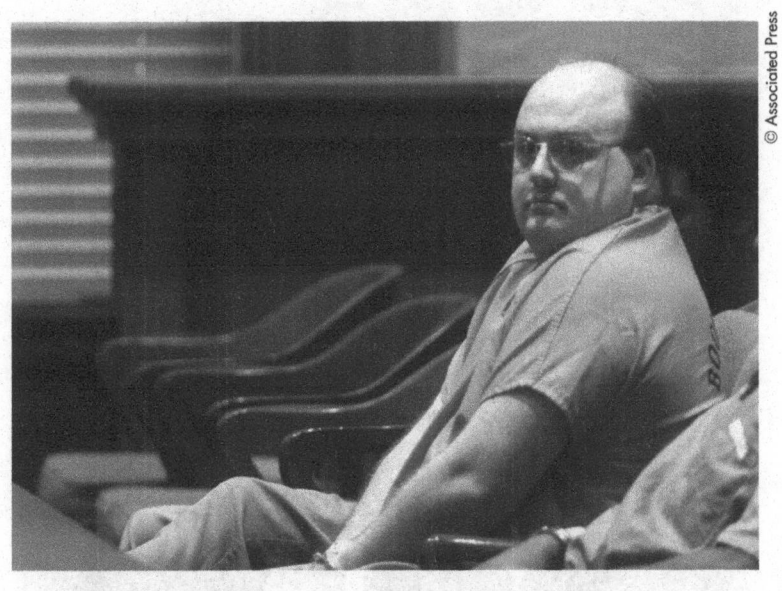

Richard Williams awaits arraignment July 22, 2002, at the Boone County (MO) Circuit Court. Williams was ultimately released when the case against him fell apart because tests that led to the charges were flawed.

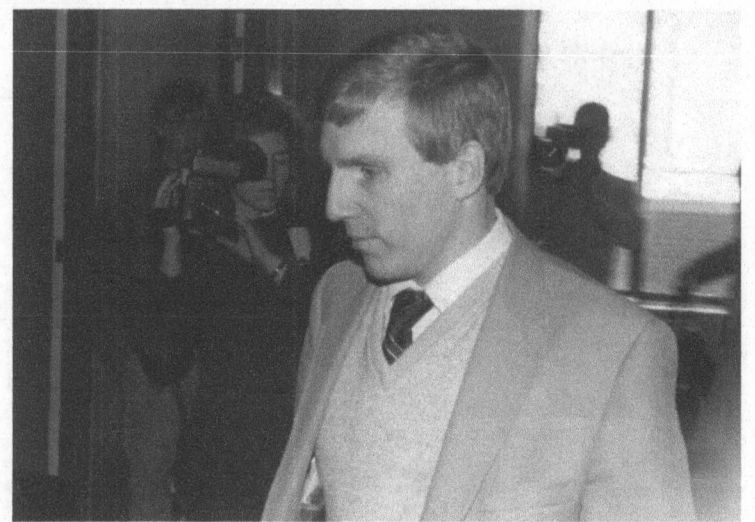

Michael Swango

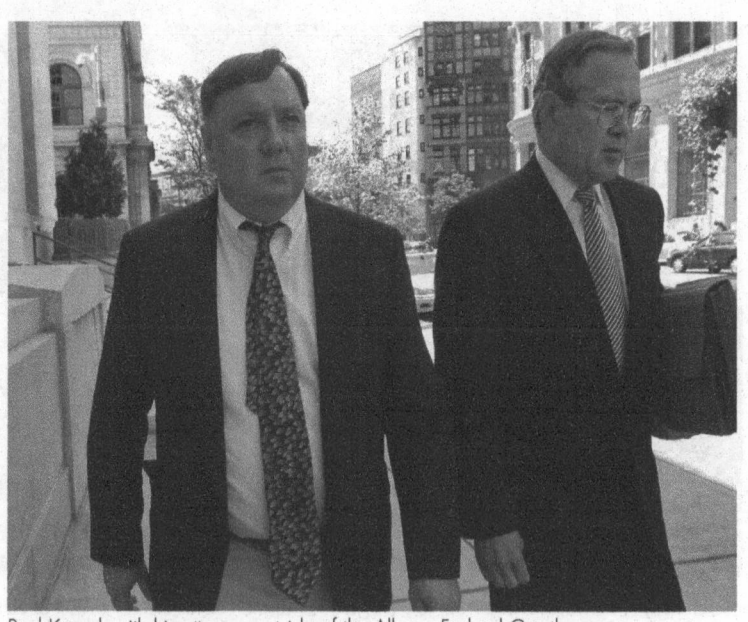

Paul Kornak with his attorney outside of the Albany Federal Courthouse.

CHAPTER 24

Busted

"You shall not murder."

—EXODUS 20:13

By now, I had a clear picture of the roadblocks that lay before us in pursuit of justice for these veterans. Nothing was more important to me than that. I sought justice for the men and women who had served their country in countless ways.

I chose someone who I felt confident would uncover all the facts and would not be deterred by those roadblocks that surface during a case of this magnitude. I reached out for Jeff Hughes, the special agent in charge of the Newark, New Jersey, office who had done such solid work in getting the Gilbert case off the ground. He directed two relatively new special agents, Gerard Poto and Kevin Russell, to conduct what was mainly a paper chase backed up by interviews with the families of victims. There would be no creepy exhumations in damp cemeteries, no grisly autopsies in freezing morgues and

215

no use of the Rieders' machine to search for traces of deadly drugs in the tissues identified by Doctor Baden.

As our second winter in freezing Albany was about to roll in on us, Kornak was indicted on October 30, 2003, by a federal grand jury for making false statements, mail fraud, wire fraud, involuntary manslaughter, and criminally negligent homicide. There was a total of forty-eight counts in all.

The indictment was somewhat complicated to read because it detailed the fraud committed in each scientific study. It reflected the incredibly difficult job Jeff Hughes and the rest of the team had connecting the dots and making sense of what Holland and Kornak were perpetrating. In essence, the indictment charged that Kornak (reminiscent of Swango), made a false statement in his application to work for the VA Medical Center in Albany; engaged in a scheme to defraud, which involved the use of mail and wire communications, the deprivation of his honest services; and falsified documents in connection with the participation of patients in clinical trials for drugs and treatments.

The indictment charged Kornak with manslaughter for causing the death of an Air Force veteran named James DiGeorgio.

What Kornak was purposely ignoring and covering up with falsified documentation was that DiGeorgio's actual blood test revealed impaired kidney and liver function. He should not have been administered the "chemotherapeutic drugs docetaxel, cisplatin, and 5-FU in connection with the TAX 325 protocol on or about May 31, 2001, and died as a result thereof on or about June 11, 2001." I had hoped for a murder charge. I wanted Kornak rotting away in a cell next to Swango, but manslaughter was a breakthrough in the fight against MSKs because it indicated Kornak knew what he was doing could kill the patient and he did not care. He wasn't a mercy killer, he was a greedy researcher advancing his own career at the cost of innocent lives.

I was so proud of my team and the detectives and scientists who backed up my intuition that we could prove more than a con game going on at Stratton. It was not a game of three-card monte. It was a murder plan.

At the news conference announcing the indictment, reporters hammered away about Doctor Holland, Kornak's boss. The media questioned Holland's complicity. What was his role, did anyone else in the VA know what was going on, should they have known? Kornak's attorney, in an argument straight out of the Nuremberg war trials, claimed that Kornak was merely part of a team and had only taken orders from Doctor Holland.

Believe me, I was not happy that Holland appeared, for the time being, to have escaped any condemnation at all. I was mad enough at him for just letting Kornak wear a white coat and ID card identifying him as a full-fledged doctor. The fact is that it was Kornak's name all over the medical reports and applications, and it was Kornak who recruited the veterans.

Soon after Kornak's indictment, a medical researcher by the name of Ann Campbell was sentenced in US District Court in Birmingham, Alabama, to fifty-seven months in prison, and fined 557,251 dollars by a federal judge for falsifying data relating to a number of persons participating in a new drug trial. She submitted the falsified data to the company that sponsored the drug study to determine the safety and effectiveness of a new drug. She was also ordered to make restitution to the company in the amount of 925,774 dollars. Those kinds of prosecutions were done before we nailed Kornak. Researchers had been found guilty of fraud, but charging a researcher with murder, like we charged Kornak, was the first ever in federal court.

About one year after the indictment of Kornak in late October 2004, about two years after the investigation began, the Food and Drug Administration posted a letter on its web site entitled, "Notice of Initiation of Disqualification Proceedings and Opportunity to Explain (NIDPOE)" directed at Holland. Finally, he was catching some heat.

Dated September 22, 2004, the letter initiated disqualification proceedings against Holland for his role in the Kornak case. The letter cites the administrative inquiry conducted by the FDA from November 14, 2002, to January 3, 2003. I must say I was not overly impressed with the FDA during our investigation. The FDA's Office of Criminal Investigations assigned two agents to work with us on a part-time basis—as if they had much more important work to do. Their contributions were minimal at best. The FDA regulatory team visited the medical center as we began the investigation and we were totally open and honest with them about where we saw things going. They had access to everything. So, I never understood why it took the FDA from January 2003 to October 2004 to propose disqualification proceedings against Holland. It is beyond my comprehension. It is important to note that prior to the letter being issued, Holland was free to continue medical research wherever he wanted. But, better late than never, I guess. The letter alleged the following violations by Holland:

- Failed to personally conduct or supervise the clinical investigations;
- Delegated certain tasks to individuals not qualified to perform them;

- Failed to adequately supervise individuals to whom tasks were delegated;
- Failed to protect the rights, safety, and welfare of subjects under his care;
- Repeatedly or deliberately submitted false information to the sponsor;
- Failed to conduct the studies or ensure they were conducted according to the approved protocols; and
- Failed to maintain adequate and accurate case histories that recorded all observations and other data pertinent to the investigation on each individual.

Holland had two options on how to respond to the charges. He could enter into a consent decree in which he agreed not to conduct research for a specified period, or he could demand a hearing. He chose the hearing.

Meanwhile, Kornak decided to forgo a trial and plead guilty. The forecast was for minus three degrees in Albany the day he was set to appear in US District Court to enter his plea. The roads leading to the courthouse were sheets of ice. I was driving one of those big Ford Crown Victoria, Police Interceptors, at the time. They were front wheel drive and turning an icy corner was an adventure as the rear end only with great reluctance followed the direction of the front end. I knew cops who kept sandbags in their trunks to help maintain traction in icy conditions. That icy day, Doctor Baden was my passenger and we almost rammed a street lamp on one particularly nerve-racking turn. That would have been a headline if the two of us were seriously injured or even killed on the way to see Kornak get his due.

But despite the weather, I was confidant things would quickly heat up in the courtroom. This plea was to be a bit different than what I had experienced in the past. For the first time in my career, I attended a plea session where the judge hearing the matter was a two-hour drive away and handling the entire affair by teleconference.

The federal courthouse in Albany houses a conference room with space for about twenty people. The new huge screen television appeared out of place in a room that was designed and built in the 1930s. It was filled to capacity and uncomfortably warm as we packed in wearing our winter coats and boots. There was a large turnout of local and national media, the attorneys representing the victims in civil suits, and lastly, some family members of the victims themselves. The plea was to begin at four o'clock.; however, for almost an hour, we stood sweating while staring at Kornak sitting at the conference table and at a screen showing only the bench behind which the judge would sit. Since many of us arrived early, we were waiting about one hour until the judge finally made his appearance at 4:20 p.m.

Usually I dislike the defendants I have brought to the bar of justice for the crimes they have committed against our veterans. I feel no pity for them. But in this case, although I can't explain it or rationalize it, I actually felt a little sorry for Kornak. He committed one of the worst crimes I had the opportunity to investigate; yet I didn't feel the disgust for him that I felt for serial killers Swango and Gilbert. I stared at Kornak and listened as he quietly confessed to crimes that resulted in the death of an American hero at a VA medical center, yet I couldn't feel any hatred towards him. As he was speaking, I felt that here is a person who could never legitimately achieve any of the goals he established. I wondered if there was someone in his life he needed to impress, maybe a parent or a spouse, that drove him to fabricate an entire medical career that caused unspeakable harm.

He seemed like a pathetic soul. Until then, I thought of him as a monster, a sociopath who thought of no one but himself. Now I could not imagine him as a person who intentionally killed anyone. But I understood his disregard for the truth and his lack of conscience didn't change patients' outcomes. I knew a famous detective in New York named Joe Coffey who hunted the "Son of Sam" serial killer for a year and developed an unnatural hatred of the man. Coffey was the first detective to interview the killer after his arrest and he told me his hatred dissolved as he walked into the interrogation room and saw David Berkowitz, the killer, for the first time. Instead of a monster, he saw in front of him a pathetic vegetable of a human being that he could not find in himself to hate. My feelings about Kornak that day in the overheated conference room were the same.

On January 18, 2005, Paul Kornak pleaded guilty to one count of criminally negligent homicide, one count of mail fraud, and one count of wire fraud. He also agreed to cooperate with investigators and answer all questions regarding his role and the role of others in this matter. The judge, who would eventually sentence Kornak, was himself a veteran who served two tours in Vietnam as an infantry officer. The sentencing was set for the end of May and in the interim, Kornak was set free but under the supervision of the U.S. Probation and Parole Office.

About one month later, Kornak's lawyer told the *New York Times* there was a "clear systems failure" at Stratton, permitting a research culture where "rules weren't followed, protocols weren't applied, and supervision was nonexistent."

I remember reading that in an article by reporter Deborah Sontag at my desk when I was back in New York City. It contained a moving interview with the widow of another veteran, Carl M. Steubing, a Battle of the Bulge veteran, who died in one of Kornak's studies. It provided a description of the killer's MO detailed by my team.

Steubing was a retired music teacher and wedding photographer, active in his church choir and an avid golfer and fisherman. He was to all who knew him an all-around terrific friend and neighbor, a genuine American hero. According to the *New York Times,* he was married to a woman twenty-four years his junior and they had seven children and three grandchildren between them. But at seventy-eight years old, he was suffering from cancer. As a man determined to live every moment of his life to the fullest, after hearing about an experimental drug treatment program at Stratton, he jumped in with both feet. Maybe it would give him a few more years to enjoy that wonderful family.

Steubing and his wife, Jayne, met Kornak together. His widow told the *New York Times* that Kornak said Steubing was "just a perfect specimen," with the body of a man half his age.

What my investigative team could prove was that Kornak knew at the time that Steubing's previous cancer and poor kidney function made him ineligible to participate in the study.

"It kills me to think that the VA system deceived us," Jayne Steubing told the reporter. "You see these youngsters at Walter Reed now," referring to the wounded coming home from Iraq, "and everybody's raving about the care they get. Well, Carl was one of these kids once, with a Bronze Star and a Purple Heart. And at the end of his life, his treatment was the antithesis of what you see on TV. It was such a betrayal."

In May of 2005, Kornak was sentenced to six years in prison. At his sentencing, he cried he was a scapegoat. He said he was being blamed for all the problems at Stratton that were eventually exposed by my investigation. Kornak could not claim he did not benefit from those problems. He was hired despite a former felony conviction and treated as a doctor despite flunking out of medical school. The revelations of the case triggered Congress to act on reforms at the VA, especially in the field of human research, that remain in place today. My hope is that these reforms are working.

Holland never went to prison. The last word on him was that, incredibly, he was working in cancer research in Georgia.

The family of James DiGeorgio, the Air Force veteran whom Kornak was convicted of killing, received a five hundred-thousand-dollar settlement from the US government.

CHAPTER 25

Legacy

"The purpose of life is a life of purpose."

—ROBERT BYRNE

As I write this memoir, I look back on my career with mixed emotions. I think about that call from Stony Brook, which threw my entire career in a direction I could never have predicted, and I am proud that I stepped up to the plate. Recently I had dinner with a psychiatrist who is the chair of the psychiatric department at a prestigious New York City hospital and was a student at Stony Brook University Medical School. We talked about the Swango case and I expressed my never-ending befuddlement about how the killer was ever accepted into the school in the first place. He told me that the Stony Brook residency program always had trouble attracting applicants because of its rural location out in Suffolk County. He said there was historically an imbalance of foreign applicants, and so when the blond-haired ex-Marine applied, administration rushed to sign him up. I had heard that before and always considered it a pathetic excuse in a profession of life and death.

He emphasized that the Swango case had a profound effect on medical credentialing. After Swango, hospitals began scrupulously checking the backgrounds of new physicians, making certain there were no unexplained gaps on their résumés regarding education or employment. Now the process takes about four months to complete. He gave me the credit for that, so on the whole, my evening ended on a high note.

Then, a few days later, reality hit me in the face with a headline in *USA Today* blaring, "VA knowingly hired doctors accused of malpractice." The article detailed the case of neurosurgeon John Henry Schneider, who had a résumé that included "more than a dozen malpractice claims and settlements in two states, Montana and Wyoming."

According to the article, some of the claims accused him of surgical mistakes that left patients maimed, paralyzed, or dead. He was accused of costing one patient bladder and bowel control after placing spinal screws incorrectly. Another time, the article reports, a patient was left paralyzed from the waist down after a device was improperly placed in his spinal canal. After another surgical patient died, the state of Wyoming revoked Schneider's medical license.

Now, this was not Swango, Gilbert, Williams, or Kornak at work. There is no indication that Schneider was a pathological serial killer using his operating room as a killing ground. The article does not allege he was a murderer.

But there is a connection to my personal rogue's gallery of MSKs: After Schneider lost his credentials in Wyoming, he applied for a job at the Iowa City VA Health Care System. I was dumbstruck when I read he was hired there. Wasn't that red flag large enough to cover the infield at Yankee Stadium?

In less than a year after Schneider started work at a hospital that serves 184,000 veterans in fifty counties in Iowa, Illinois, and Missouri, some of his patients started suffering severe complications, according to the *USA Today* article.

The newspaper cited a case in which Schneider performed four brain surgeries in four weeks on a sixty-five-year-old veteran who subsequently died. Clearly somebody was watching and blew the whistle loud enough for *USA Today* to hear and take some action.

Even more frightening is that the newspaper found Schneider's circumstances were not an isolated case. The story goes on to report that a VA medical center in Oklahoma knowingly hired a psychiatrist who had been sanctioned for sexual misconduct and subsequently slept with a patient. The newspaper cited more cases.

As a result of the reporter's brilliant work, the VA determined the hiring of Schneider in Iowa City…and potentially that of an unknown number of doctors…was illegal." Federal law bars the agency from hiring physicians whose licenses have been revoked by a state board, even if they still hold an active license in another state. I guess I need to add another red flag. *Do Not Hire a Doctor Whose License Has Been Revoked.*

Around the world the situation appears even worse. Hardly a day goes by that we don't see a newspaper headline about a doctor or nurse accused of being an MSK.

In June 2017, Canadian Nurse Elizabeth Wettlaufer was sentenced to life in prison for killing eight elderly patients with lethal insulin doses. She apologized profusely at her sentencing, crying as she admitted causing "tremendous pain and suffering and death." She said she was extremely sorry.

The judge saw right through her. "It is a complete betrayal of trust when a caregiver does not prolong life but terminates it. She was not an angel of mercy; she was the shadow of death that passed over them on the night shift where she supervised."

I understand we will never see the end of these cases as we will never see the end of serial killers who stalk the streets of Anytown USA. Until we find a way to short-circuit whatever that is in their brains that makes them kill, all we can do is try to catch them sooner better than later.

When Paul Kornak pleaded guilty in January 2005, I was criticized by some colleagues for being overly emotional at a news conference about the case. I remember being very charged up about the success we had and a little outraged that Kornak's boss, Doctor James Holland, was one with whom we still must deal. (He eventually got five years' probation and a 502,925-dollar judgment.) But I was also trying to hide my private angst over my decision to retire in May. "Would this be my last hurrah?" I wondered.

On the train ride back to New York, I experienced the typical self-doubt of someone voluntarily giving up a lifetime of work. I explored whether I had any long-lasting impact on the giant-sized bureaucracy to which I devoted more than three decades. By the time I reached Grand Central Terminal, my answer was *Yes!*

There was no doubt in my mind that I was leaving the agency much better equipped to handle the Swangos and Gilberts that were sure to show up in the future. I paved the way for my successors to exploit a powerful network of top medical forensic professionals throughout the world. Many of the fresh-faced new agents I hired were now supervisors, well versed in the RFPs.

My boss did not want me to retire, but he acknowledged there was a second career out there that would pay me well and allow me to continue the work I started that day in the small dorm room at Northport.

My successful medical serial killer cases brought a great amount of positive publicity to the VA OIG and greatly enhanced its reputation in the entire law enforcement community. No other OIG had made cases like these and my agent friends would even tell me the FBI was envious of some of these successes. Even before my retirement was official, I was invited to speak at an FBI serial killer conference along with many other nationally recognized serial killer experts. The positive recognition by the FBI after all those years felt very rewarding.

I knew I would continue to lecture and be available to consult in future cases. Sitting at a pool in Florida with nothing but memories would not be satisfying for me. I had to stay involved. So nowadays, with the thermometer stuck around twenty degrees or bursting at ninety-five degrees at 6:11 a.m., I can be found standing on the platform of the Hicksville, New York, train station awaiting the Long Island Railroad into Manhattan's Penn Station. I'm not alone; there is plenty of gray hair on the train with me.

I continue my life as a medical center investigator, interviewing doctors, nurses, and other hospital employees suspected of wrongdoing; attending hearings; presenting my findings to prosecutors; and working with law enforcement. I've become particularly fond of working with the Office of the Special Narcotics Prosecutor for the City of New York in combating drug diversion. In a recent case, my efforts resulted in the arrest and conviction of a director of pharmacy for stealing more than two hundred thousand doses of oxycodone. This case made the papers as far away as New Zealand.

I am also busy presenting my fraud awareness briefings to hospital staff, and of course, my Red Flag Protocols to law enforcement and nursing groups throughout the world. I like to keep my hands in both teaching and investigating. George Bernard Shaw wrote, "Those who can, do; those who can't, teach." I'm not sure I agree 100 percent with that but I feel in order to stay on the cutting edge of investigations. I need to do both.

Helping me a great deal with that challenge is my role as the president of the Society of Professional Investigators in New York City. This is an organization founded in 1956 by NYPD detectives and agents of the Office of Strategic Services (OSS), the precursor to the CIA. Its members are a unique collection of experienced detectives from just about any law enforcement agency you can imagine.

On a perfect June 1994 day, the fiftieth anniversary of D-Day, I was fortunate to sit in a sky booth at Yankee Stadium with my wife, Eileen, my daughter Allison, and my son Jonathan, along with the families of five other World War II veterans who were going to be honored that day.

The vets were brought on the field and introduced one by one as veterans of the Normandy invasion. One of those American heroes was my father, Staff Sgt. Alan Sackman of the 628th Tank Destroyer Battalion. The standing room only-crowd gave the vets a Yankee Stadium standing ovation befitting Derek Jeter, as manager Joe Torre presented each vet a plaque and offered a heartfelt handshake. It was a wonderful event and I will forever be grateful to the Yankee organization for this day.

One of the vets also honored that day was U.S. Army paratrooper Joseph Beyrle, who had been captured by the Germans, escaped, and fought with the Russian army until the end of the war. His son, John Beyrle, became U.S. ambassador to the Russian Federation.

I hope my dedication and my decades of hard work are an expression of my thanks to the men and women who have fought so hard and sacrificed so much for our freedom. These thoughts remained constant during my tenure at the VA Office of Inspector General. It remained my guiding principle through twenty-five years of criminal investigations helping veterans and the VA.

Each year, the Society of Professional Investigators honors our wounded warriors at an annual dinner. In 2017, we honored retired US Army Captain Florent Groberg, a Congressional Medal of Honor recipient. It makes the event a very special occasion.

There have been improvements in identifying and prosecuting MSKs. Whistle-blower protection is the best it has ever been. The Red Flags Protocol have been shared courtesy of my writing, the internet, and my public speaking. Hopefully one day, this will be a topic only for the history books.

ACKNOWLEDGMENTS

Without the help of some very special people, this book would never have become more than some notes scribbled on a napkin over a lunch shared by the authors.

We must thank the men and women of the US Department of Veterans Affairs who every day work tirelessly to honor their mission of serving our nation's heroes: the special agents, auditors, and medical professionals of the Veterans Affairs Office of the Inspector General (VA OIG) who utilize their special skills to help keep veterans, VA programs, facilities, and operations safe, secure, and free of fraud, waste, and abuse. Particularly former VA OIG special agents Thomas Valery, Samantha Lockery, Steve Plante, John McDermott, Robert Franco, Michael Seitler, and Donna Neves. Special Agent Jeffrey Hughes, who worked both the Gilbert and Kornak cases, is now the Assistant Inspector General for Investigations in Washington, D.C., and there are so many more.

Essential to our work are the forensic nurses who bridge the gap between physicians and law enforcement personnel to successfully investigate suspicious medical events. Particularly VA nurses Mary Sullivan, Linda Delong, and Shirley Henley.

Prosecutors like William Welch, Gary Brown, Joseph Conway, and Grant Jaquith who were not afraid to tackle the most difficult medical serial killer (MSK) cases.

Doctor Michael Baden, the world's greatest forensic pathologist, who taught an entire federal agency how to investigate medical serial killers.

Retired FBI toxicologist and Special Agent Brian Donnelly, whose scientific and investigative skills are second to none, made much of our success possible.

Also, the National Medical Services, particularly Doctor Michael Rieders, for always finding time to answer questions about the science involved with catching MSKs.

We would have nothing without the love and support of our families and closest friends:

Eileen Sackman, Allison Sackman Matos, and Jonathan Sackman. Lenor Romano, Andrew Vecchione, Brian Vecchione, and Suzanne Vecchione. Emily Schmetterer, Morty Matz, and Annette Georgious.

Without the extraordinary effort of our agent, Frank Weimann, and his assistant, Sanali Chanchani, and our attorney, Dino Amoroso, the incredible story of Bruce Sackman's work in bringing down Medical Serial Killers could not have been told.

Special thanks as always to our friend and colleague Doctor Sheldon Shuch, PhD, who teaches teachers how to teach and readers how to read, and who loves a good story well told.

ABOUT THE AUTHORS

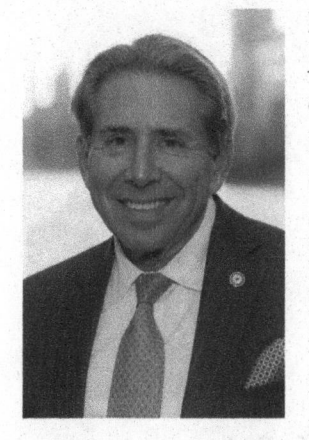 **Bruce Sackman** served as the Special Agent in Charge, U.S. Department of Veteran Affairs (VA), Office of Inspector General, Criminal Investigations Division, Northeast Field Office until May 2005 when he retired after thirty-two years of service. In this capacity, he was responsible for all major criminal investigations involving the VA from West Virginia to Maine. During his tenure, he was involved in hundreds of investigations involving allegations of fraud, corruption, false claims, thefts, patient assaults, pharmaceutical drug diversions, and suspicious hospital deaths. He was also responsible for supervising the successful investigation of the nation's first homicide conviction in connection with pharmaceutical research. His cases have been featured on the Discovery Health Channel, CNN, MSNBC, *America's Most Wanted*, and on Home Box Office. He is the recipient of many awards for his investigations and for his efforts in encouraging the profession of forensic nursing. Sackman has lectured at several forensic-related conferences, state police organizations, the Federal Law Enforcement Training Center, universities, and medical related symposia.

Sackman is self-employed as a licensed private investigator in New York City specializing in healthcare-related matters. Under contract, he directs all major investigations for a major New York metropolitan regional healthcare system. He is president of the Society of Professional Investigators in New York City and serves on the board of directors of the American Academy for Professional Law Enforcement.

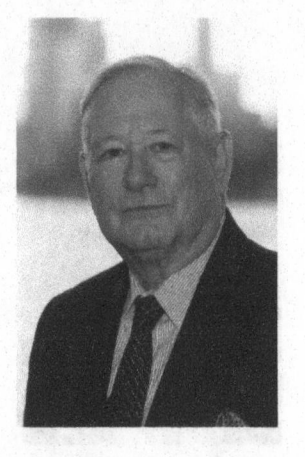

Jerry Schmetterer is an award-winning print and broadcast journalist. *Behind the Murder Curtain* is his sixth nonfiction book. He is a former bureau chief and editor at the *NY Daily News* and managing editor at CNN and WPIX in New York. He served for twelve years as spokesman for the Brooklyn District Attorney's Office. He is past president of the NY Press Club and currently serves as a Trustee. He lives in Manhattan with his wife, Emily.

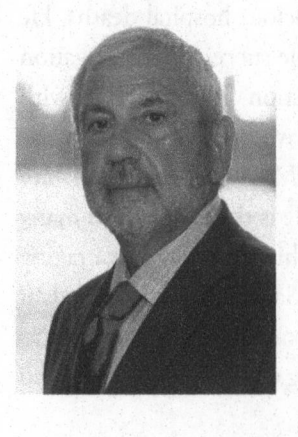

Michael Vecchione is a former Chief of the Rackets Division of the Brooklyn District Attorney's Office, topping off a career of forty years as a prosecutor. *Behind the Murder Curtain* is his third nonfiction book. He is a frequent contributor to true crime television productions as an expert on organized crime. He lives in Long Island City, NY, with his partner, Lenor Romano.